VETERINARY DENTISTRY
for the
small animal technician

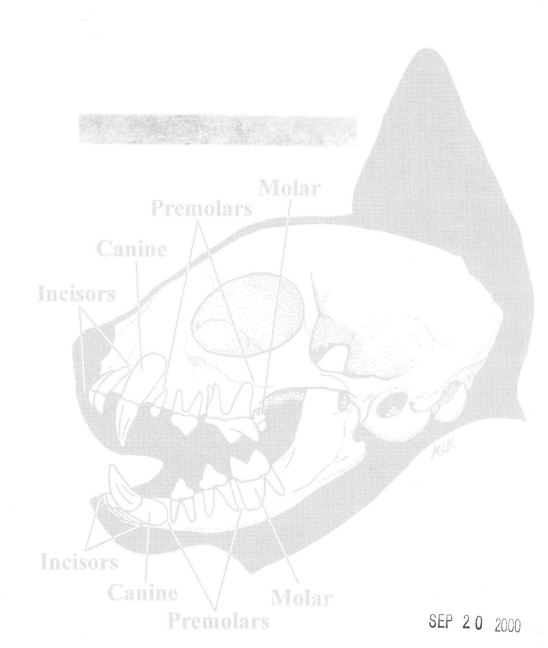

Molar

Premolars

Canine

Incisors

Incisors

Canine

Molar

Premolars

RELATED BOOKS
by
Iowa State University Press

An Atlas of Veterinary Dental Radiology
Donald H. DeForge and
Benjamin H. Colmery III, editors, 2000

The Practice of Veterinary Dentistry:
A Team Effort
Jan Bellows, 1999

Self-Assessment Color Review of
Veterinary Dentistry
Frank J. M. Verstraete, editor, 1999

Manual of Small Animal Dentistry,
Second Edition
David A. Crossley and Susanna Penman,
editors, 1995

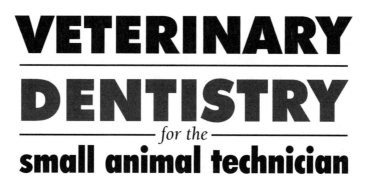

VETERINARY
DENTISTRY
for the
small animal technician

M. Lynne Kesel DVM

*with illustrations by M. Lynne Kesel DVM
and Anna Kendall*

Iowa State University Press / Ames

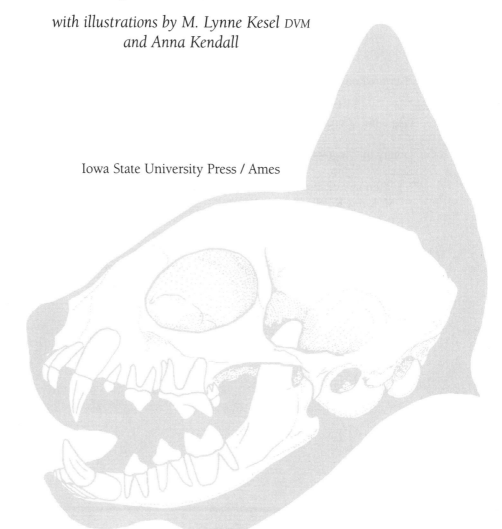

M. Lynne Kesel DVM is an associate professor in the Department of Clinical Sciences at Colorado State University. Since 1989, she has been in charge of the clinical Small Animal Dentistry Service at the university's Veterinary Teaching Hospital.

Iowa State University Press
2121 South State Avenue, Ames, Iowa 50014

Orders: 1-800-862-6657
Office: 1-515-292-0140
Fax: 1-515-292-3348
Web site: www.isupress.edu

⊛ Printed on acid-free paper in the United States of America

First edition, 2000

Library of Congress Cataloging-in-Publication Data
Kesel, M. Lynne
    Veterinary dentistry for the small animal technician / M. Lynne Kesel; with illustrations by
    M. Lynne Kesel and Anna Kendall. — 1st ed.
        p. cm.
    Includes bibliographical references (p.) and index.
    ISBN 0-8138-2037-5
    1. Veterinary dentistry. 2. Dogs—Diseases. 3. Cats—Diseases. I. Title.
SF867 .K47 2000
636.7'08976—dc21   00-024450

The last digit is the print number: 9   8   7   6   5   4   3   2   1

For

Martha, Anna, and Shaela

Contents

Preface

Early in 1997, Dr. Bernie Rollin suggested I write this book. He and I had previously collaborated in coediting a major reference work in the laboratory animal field for which we had both written chapters. Since beginning our project in the two-volume work *The Experimental Animal in Biomedical Research,* I had changed jobs in the university from laboratory animal medicine and was teaching veterinary students in clinical rotations involving routine surgeries and small animal dentistry. When Bernie said I should get busy and write a dental book for veterinarians, I smugly quashed the notion, pointing out that there were several excellent books recently published or being published on that topic. And then he said, "How about a book on dentistry for technicians?" The complete lack of books on the subject and my interest made it a natural.

Small animal dentistry is, I feel, one area of veterinary medicine in which technicians can act like nurse-practitioners in the human field. The nurse-practitioner is highly trained (to the level of a physician) in one limited area. He or she does not have the in-depth, general education of a physician or see the complete range of rotations that a physician in training would. The nurse-practitioner works with a physician, uses the physician's wider knowledge and experience as a resource, and knows when to refer problems to the physician. For instance, the nurse-midwife would seek a physician's guidance if a pregnant patient showed signs of a heart condition.

In this book, I have attempted to explain even fairly complicated dental procedures so that the technician can understand what is being done and how to assist, but not necessarily how to do them. In veterinary medicine, technicians have been taught how to administer anesthetics and even how to perform routine surgeries to free veterinarians for other tasks. Depending on the jurisdiction this may be perfectly legal as long as the veterinarian provides supervision. There are some areas where the law severely limits the role of anyone except the licensed veterinarian in providing service. Often, this has evolved because of abuses in the system (e.g., the veterinarian takes a day off, and the technicians do the surgery). The technician should always be aware of the legal limits of his or her job and refuse to perform unlawfully. If something should go wrong, there is always the possibility of being named in a lawsuit and losing a technician license and/or money for damages.

The American Veterinary Dental College has published thorough guidelines describing who should provide veterinary dental care (see Appendix 3). To stay within these suggested guidelines for technicians is always safe. If a veterinarian expects the technician to exceed these guidelines (which is very common), it is worth consulting local or regional technician organizations or even the state board of veterinary medicine. In some areas, the response will be "Whatever the veterinarian asks of the technician is legal as long as he or she is supervised by the veterinarian."

Many veterinary schools still do not have dental specialists on staff to teach veterinary students about dentistry, and technicians who have learned only the material in Chapters 1, 4, and 5 may well have more knowledge about anatomy, periodontal disease, and cleaning teeth than their bosses! Because I have attempted to present information in an accessible manner, technicians who have purchased this book may want to loan it to their veterinarians; veterinarians may want to purchase it for their technicians. (I hope so!)

In the final analysis, the technician is providing an invaluable service to pets and their owners even if limited to dental prophies (cleanings) and client education. In most cases, home and professional dental care can ward off periodontal disease and its potential ramifications, which can be painful, debilitating, and even life threatening.

Acknowledgments

First among many, I would like to thank my dear friends Bernard Rollin and Vicki Matteson, who read the manuscript chapter by chapter as it came out of my printer. They faced a daunting task: attempting to make my prose intelligible when I wandered off the path with run-on sentences or bizarre ways of expressing myself, as well as cleaning up my spelling and occasional grammatical lapses. Any errors in style or substance still belong to me, however, since I had the final word at the keyboard as I decided whether to accept their improvements (I gratefully accepted most). Bernie also was my goad to write this book in the first place, and Vicki was my inspiration as a technician par excellence.

I want to thank my dental mentor, Dr. Ed Eisner, for the knowledge he has imparted to me over the years and for the photographs of cases he shared for this book. Most of the other photographs in the book were taken by Jenger Smith or Charles Kerlee of the Colorado State University Photo Lab. They also "duped" slides for me and scanned illustrations, and all of their help is very appreciated.

My daughter Anna Kendall aided me not only by producing highly detailed drawings but also with manipulation of computer images of the illustrations, and to her I say, "Thanks, babe."

VETERINARY
DENTISTRY
for the
small animal technician

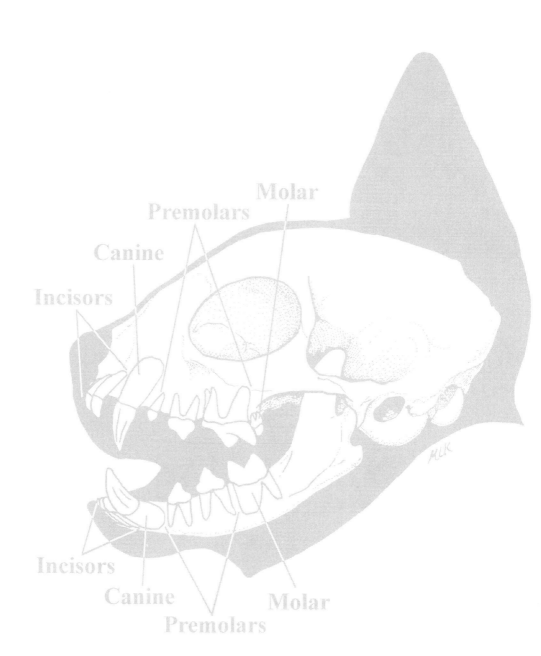

chapter 1

Oral and Dental Functional Anatomy

By tradition as well as necessity, a text must begin with the basics. A mechanic could not fix a car effectively if he did not understand the layout and appearance of the engine (the anatomy) or the way it should work (the physiology). A surgeon would be ineffective, and probably dangerous, if she or he ignored the importance of understanding the anatomy and physiology of the structures she or he was intending to alter by surgery. So it is with you, the veterinary dental technician. You should have an understanding of oral and dental structures and how they work in health as well as illness. With this knowledge, you can be a full participant in the total health care of the patient. Understanding begins with knowing about the formation of teeth in the jaw (Fig. 1-1).

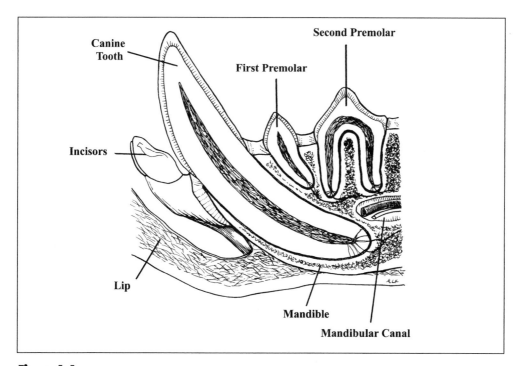

Figure 1-1

Diagrammatic representation of the rostral mandible of a dog. The lip, canine tooth, and the first and second premolars are shown in a cutaway view to demonstrate the relationship of the teeth to each other, the periodontal tissues, and the mandibular canal. The incisors rostral to the canine are not shown as a sectioned view.

THE EMBRYOLOGY OF THE TOOTH

To grossly simplify embryology, which is a complex and fascinating subject, we can speak of three basic tissues that are transformed into all of the organs and structures of the animal: the ectoderm, mesoderm, and endoderm. The ectoderm is the layer on the outside of the early embryo, which will eventually become epithelium (skin), as well as other things (like the enamel of teeth). The association of tooth enamel with the epithelium is important because something that can affect one may affect the other. For instance, before it became rare due to widespread vaccination, canine distemper caused enamel deficits in dogs who were infected as puppies because the virus has a tropism for (attraction to) epithelial cells such as the ameloblast, the enamel-producing cell. When the ameloblast is actively producing enamel for a tooth and it is infected by the virus, it stops functioning, and there will be no enamel on the tooth surface where that cell was situated. Severe fevers during tooth development can cause damage to the enamel organ (the collective name for all the ameloblasts making the enamel of a tooth crown) as well, just as they can cause the loss of hair follicles in the skin by killing those cells.

The mesoderm is the middle tissue of the early embryo. It will become the bones, muscles, and most of the solid organs (like the liver and kidneys) of the animal. It also forms the major part of the tooth, the dentin.

The endoderm is the third early embryonic tissue. It forms the heart and blood vessels. Since teeth have a blood supply in their pulp, it could be said that teeth are unique in having components of all three types of tissues.

The ectoderm, or epithelium, initiates the formation of a "tooth bud." In the place where a tooth will develop, the epithelium invaginates (pokes) into the mesoderm, or mesothelium, of the tissue that will become bone (Fig. 1-2A). The process is much like pushing your finger into a flaccid water balloon; as the wall of the balloon "invaginates" into the water, it forms a tunnel. As the tunnel that will become the tooth bud gets deeper in the mesothelium, it flares out and then acts as if it were pushed up in the middle of the point (Fig. 1-2B). Eventually it forms a double-walled, roughly bell-shaped structure in the outline of the crown of the tooth (the crown is the portion of the tooth that will be covered with enamel and erupted into the mouth). The formation of this crown-shaped bell induces mesothelial cells inside it (a bud-shaped bit of tissue known as the dental papilla) to differentiate into odontoblasts, which will make dentin, the main structural component of the tooth. Simultaneously, epithelial cells adjacent to the odontoblasts are induced to become ameloblasts, which will make enamel. The rest of the "bell" becomes support cells for the ameloblasts; the entire epithelial complex is referred to as the enamel organ.

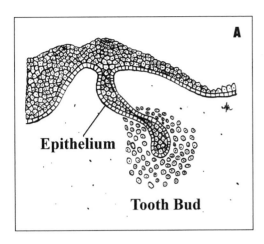

Figure 1-2

Initial formation of the tooth bud.

(A) The appearance of the invagination of ectodermal cells (epithelium) into the mesoderm is the first stage of a developing tooth. The presence of the ectoderm is stimulating the concentration of mesodermal cells that will eventually form the dentin of the tooth.

(B) The bell-shaped cup of the tooth bud is beginning to take shape. The depression in the middle of the tip is where the crown of the tooth will form.

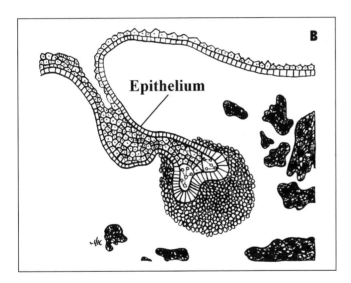

The growth of the tooth begins at the tip of the crown and progresses toward the root. The growth of the enamel organ ceases when the crown has reached its full length and enamel thickness, but dentin continues to be laid down as the root develops. Once the enamel is fully formed, the tooth will begin to erupt with the root unfinished. If the tooth is a primary, or deciduous ("baby"), tooth, it will be replaced by a secondary or permanent tooth. When the primary tooth bud is formed, the epithelial cells form a secondary tooth bud, which will remain dormant until it is time for the permanent tooth to replace the primary one (Fig. 1-3).

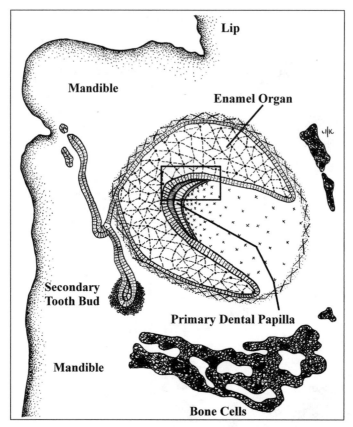

Figure 1-3

An active enamel organ/tooth bud. Enamel and dentin are beginning to form at the tip of the future tooth crown. When enough enamel and dentin are mineralized, the arrow-head-shaped tooth crowns will be visible on X rays of pups in utero. Imaging of tooth buds at this later stage signals that a pup is mature enough to survive outside the uterus.

FORMATION OF THE ROOT

There is no enamel on the surface of the root. Instead a structure called Hertwig's epithelial root sheath takes over the growth of the root. It starts as a band around the tooth at the base of the crown (or more than one band at the base of the crown in a multiple-rooted tooth). Hertwig's sheath is the source of the cementocytes that produce the partially mineralized surface of the root, called cementum. Odontoblasts multiply at the apical (root side) edge of Hertwig's sheath, lengthening the root as they form dentin. This formation of root dentin pushes the crown toward the surface of the jaw through the bone. This is necessary to allow the root to lengthen within the limited width of the jaw. Hertwig's epithelial root sheath stays essentially in the same position while the root lengthens and the tooth erupts. It ceases to

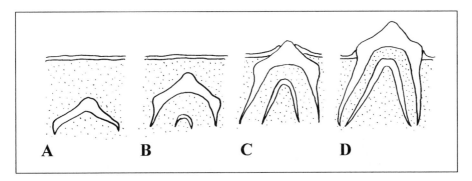

Figure 1-4

The development of the tooth from deep in the bone.

(A) The tooth crown is first evident.

(B) Once the crown is complete, the root starts to grow, forcing the crown toward the surface of the jaw.

(C) The root is still lengthening when the tooth breaks through the gingiva.

(D) The roots are full-length and are beginning to constrict at the apex. Note that the growing portion of the root stays in the same place while the tooth crown moves.

function when the root tip, or apex, is formed. As the growth of the root reaches its predetermined length, the sheath constricts until only a tiny opening for blood supply and nerves is left (Fig. 1-4).

This process is called apexification (for the formation of the apex of the root), and it has important implications for the pulp inside the tooth. A tooth will not erupt further if the tooth has apexified, which is a condition found in impacted teeth, where something mechanically obstructs eruption, partially or completely.

FORMATION OF ENAMEL

Enamel is the hardest tissue produced by a living thing; it exceeds the hardness of coral. The ameloblasts secrete the enamel matrix toward the odontoblasts, and the body of the ameloblast cell is thereby moved away from the dentin of the tooth. Enamel is composed almost entirely of mineral in crystallized prisms that are lined up at right angles to the surface of the tooth. When enamel is broken or chipped, it will typically do so in these right angles, following these prisms all the way to the surface of the dentin, rather than across the enamel surface (Fig. 1-5). The enamel of teeth is intended to act as a deterrent to wear and as a cover for dentinal tubules (see below), but it is very brittle. It is therefore typically very thin, usually a millimeter or less in thickness when mature, regardless of species.

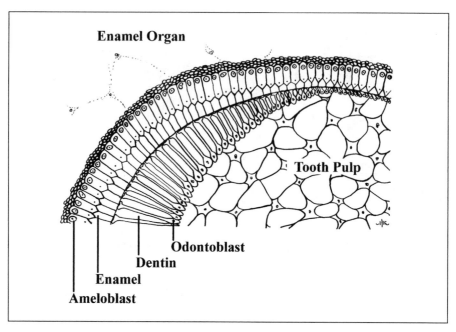

Figure 1-5

Detail of Figure 1-3. The tip of the tooth crown shows the cell bodies of the ameloblasts forming enamel prisms. Adjacent to the prisms are the ends of the processes of the odontoblasts. Dentin is being formed between the processes of the odontoblasts, and the cell bodies of the odontoblasts reside next to the rest of the tooth pulp, the cells of which provide nourishment for the odontoblasts.

FORMATION OF DENTIN

Odontoblasts are modified bone cells. The minerals they secrete (called calcium hydroxy-apatite) are mostly calcium and are similar in makeup to that of enamel and bone. The main difference in the three is how the material is laid down and how much organic (nonmineral, or soft) material it contains. The odontoblast, like the ameloblast, secretes its product toward the enamel/dentin interface. The body of the odontoblast retreats away from this surface toward the middle of the tooth. It forms a layer with other odontoblasts along the boundary of the soft tissue center of the tooth called the tooth pulp. During this retreat, the odontoblasts leave a threadlike process of cytoplasm behind within a tubule formed of dentin; the dentin from adjacent odontoblasts joins to form a solid dentinal wall perforated by dentinal tubules. Dentinal tubules extend nearly to the surface of the dentin/enamel interface (or the dentin/cementum interface of the root), and they allow fluid exchange within the dentin of the tooth as long as the odontoblast is alive. Therefore dentin is a live tissue. Enamel is not a live tissue since no part of a live cell stays within it.

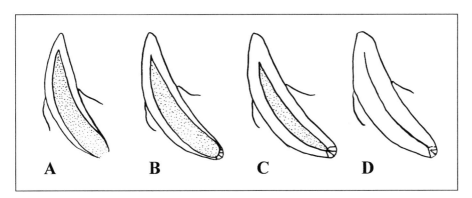

Figure 1-6

Root and pulp development and aging.

(A) A recently erupted canine tooth of a dog, age six months. The apex has not closed (apexified), and a wide-open pulp is surrounded by only a thin shell of dentin on the root.

(B) At approximately 14–18 months of age the canine root apex closes.

(C) A mature dog (4 to 5 years) shows the result of further deposition of dentin with age.

(D) The dentinal walls of the old dog (>10 years) are so thick that the pulp is almost nonexistent and contains little blood supply.

The dentin that is formed before the tooth erupts is called primary dentin (not to be confused with primary teeth). The dentin that completes the tooth root and continues to form as the tooth matures, causing the dentinal walls to thicken throughout life (Fig. 1-6), is the secondary dentin.

It can be seen that the odontoblasts get closer and closer together as they secrete dentin behind them toward the outside of the tooth. This may be why dentin laid down late in life is of a darker color (tan or brownish); more dentinal tubules mean more organic material, which is more likely to take up stain from the mouth.

It also may be that dentin nearer the center of the tooth has been rapidly laid down in response to a stimulus, such as wear or a closed fracture (a chip that does not enter the pulp), and therefore contains or incorporates more organic matter. Once damage has occurred to the tooth, and the protective enamel is lost from the surface, the dentinal tubules are left open to the oral environment. Since the tubules are too small to allow the ingression of bacteria, an infection does not occur, yet thermal and chemical stimuli are transmitted more readily to the nerve in the pulp. This is why when we get a "cavity" we get a sharp pain in the tooth with cold, heat, or sugar. The tooth pulp tries to cover over the open tubules by increasing the amount of dentinal "insulation" between itself and the stimulus; odontoblasts toward the stimulus are turned on, and additional mineral is laid down within the tubules. This dentin that is laid down in response to a stimulus is called tertiary dentin; it was formerly known as reparative dentin, for obvious reasons.

When a tooth is quite young, its walls are relatively thin. However, dentinal tubules are wide and contain more cell cytoplasm in the odontoblastic processes. This young tooth is more resilient because of the amount of organic material in the pulp and odontoblastic processes as well as the intracellular fluid that bathes the dentin from the processes. As the tooth ages, the blood supply becomes atretic (decreases to nonfunctional) because the pulp narrows; the cell processes are lost as tubules also are mineralized. These old teeth are not fractured as often as young teeth because old animals do not tend to abuse their teeth as much as young animals and the teeth are stronger from an increased thickness of dentin. You can appreciate this when you think of the wall of the tooth of a young animal as a single-thickness pane of glass as compared with that of an old animal, which is more like the thickness of a glass tabletop. It takes a tremendous blow to break the tabletop, whereas a sharp tap with a hard object will shatter the windowpane.

THE TOOTH PULP

The bulk of the tooth pulp is composed of blood vessels (arterial and venous capillaries), lymph vessels, and sensory nerve tissue maintained in a latticework of fibrous tissue and fibrocytes. In this way, it is similar to subcutaneous tissue without the fat cells, except that the odontoblasts are lined up on the periphery of the tooth pulp. The vessels and nerves are branches of the main vessels and nerves of the respective jaws. The blood supply supports the functioning of the odontoblasts as well as the other elements of the pulp. As in other live tissues, the sensory nerves are present to avoid damage to the pulp by noxious stimuli. An interesting fact in dogs and cats is that the apex of the tooth root completely closes over in about 80 percent of the teeth, leaving only small, sievelike microscopic openings for the vessels and nerves that enter the pulp. In humans, the apex of the tooth is constricted but is almost always formed as a canal rather than the so-called apical delta of our common pets. This has implications for endodontic therapy (see Chap. 10).

THE PERIODONTIUM

Up to this point we have ignored perhaps the most important aspect of the tooth: the tissues that support it so that it can perform its intended function. All of the tissues that come into contact with the tooth are part of the *perio-* ("around") *dontium* ("tooth"). Just as a fencepost cannot function to hold up a fence if the ground around it is soft mud, a tooth will loosen and exfoliate (fall out) if the periodontal tissues lose their integrity.

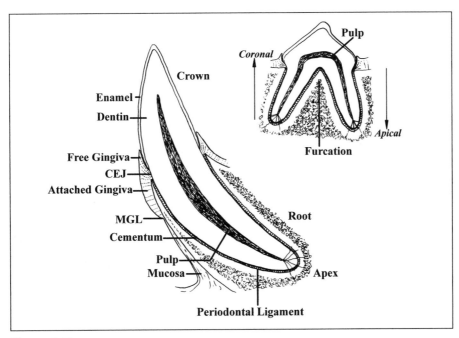

Figure 1-7
The tooth and its parts.

The most critical part of the periodontium is the periodontal ligament (Fig. 1-7). Ligaments in general are fibrous bands between bones; the tooth's dentin, of course, is a modified bone. The fibers of the periodontal ligament are lined up perpendicular to the root surface and suspend the tooth between the bone of the tooth's alveolus (the root's "socket") and the root. The fibers intermesh both with the fibers and the calcified tissue of the cementum on the tooth side and with Sharpey's fibers attached to the bone on the other. The space between the fibers of the ligament is filled with fibrocytes, blood vessels, and nerves. When we adjust how hard we bite down on something, the sensation comes from nerves in the periodontal ligament. The periodontal ligament, like all of the periodontium, has a good blood supply and is constantly renewing and repairing itself in the face of constant wear and tear.

The periodontal ligament has two functions other than sensation and holding the tooth in its socket: cushioning of forces to the tooth and separation of dentin from bone. Imagine, if you will, teeth made of glass within glass jaws, the glass of the teeth being just a little bit tougher than that of the jaws. In one case let us put a thin layer of sponge rubber between tooth and jaw, in the alveolus. In the other, we will glue the tooth to the alveolus. The process of normal chewing will cause microscopic or major fractures to the jaw with the tooth solidly attached, as opposed to cushioned. Catching a tennis ball or a flying disc will be even more likely to cause a fracture in the uncushioned model.

To understand the importance of a physical barrier between bone and dentin, we must review the physiology of normal bone. All live bone is constantly being replaced on a microscopic level. A bone cell called an osteoclast tunnels through the formed bone and, like the video character Pac Man, "eats" the calcified tissue. Right behind the osteoclast is another bone cell, an osteoblast. The osteoblast follows along the tunnel and fills it up with new bone; the structure the two create is called an osteoid seam. Dentin, since it is made of similar components to bone, could be considered a denser bone, and osteoclasts would be very happy to tunnel through it. Why they usually do not is the presence of the periodontal ligament, which acts as a barrier to osteoclasts, except in certain disease conditions (see Chaps. 4 and 10). One of the concepts important to remember here is that, unlike bone, dentin does not remodel or change once it is formed, except to lose vitality (if odontoblasts die) or to be destroyed by disease conditions such as caries ("cavities") or resorptive lesions.

The alveolar bone is the same as the bone on the surface of the jaw or any other bone. It is a dense, white cortical type of bone. Surrounding it and continuous with it is less-dense cancellous bone. In a radiograph (X ray) the dense dentin of the tooth will be the whitest part of the image, with a darker pulp present in its center. At the surface of the tooth another dark band occurs where the nonmineralized periodontal ligament lies. The alveolar bone just next to the ligament is whiter than the rest of the bone because it is on edge in the radiograph and is denser than the surrounding cancellous bone. This white line is called the lamina dura.

The continuous line of bone that supports the teeth is called the alveolar crest. This bone is dependent upon the presence of tooth roots for its existence; if teeth are never formed or if they are lost, the alveolar crest disappears, and the jaw becomes flat.

THE ATTACHED GINGIVA, GINGIVAL SULCUS, AND ORAL MUCOSA

Although the periodontal ligament gets the credit for holding the tooth in place, the attached gingiva protects the periodontal ligament from invasion by oral bacteria. The attached gingiva, commonly and inexactly called the gums, is the firm epidermal tissue that mounds up at the base of the tooth. In dogs, it can be either unpigmented (pink) or pigmented. In cats it is essentially unpigmented. The attached gingiva adheres closely to the underlying bone. If you look closely at attached gingiva (yours or an animal's), you will see pinpoint divots all over its surface. These divots are evidence of the attachment of epidermal pegs to the underside of the surface layer, which in turn are attached to the bone, like tie-downs for skin. The attached gingiva does not move over the bone, unlike the oral mucosa adjacent to it. The oral mucosa moves freely over bone or the connective tissue of the cheeks and lips and is very elastic, to allow for full opening of the mouth. Oral mucosa is not, strictly speaking, a periodontal tissue, since its loose attachment would allow bacteria to enter; it is never next to the teeth in a normal mouth. The border between the oral mucosa and the attached gingiva is sharply delineated. It is called the mucogingival line, or MGL.

The attached gingiva has a leading edge that laps over the tooth called the free gingival margin. This margin varies in width by species (it is usually a millimeter or less wide in cats, for instance) and by tooth. In most healthy dogs it ranges from about 2 to 4 mm wide. The crevice between the tooth and the free gingival margin is called the gingival sulcus. The bottom of the sulcus is formed by fibers of epithelium that adhere the attached gingiva to the tooth at the border between root and crown, otherwise known as the cemento-enamel junction, or CEJ. This is an important landmark for periodontal health, as loss of this attachment signals the beginning of periodontal destruction.

The epithelium that faces the tooth surface within the sulcus is called, not surprisingly, sulcular or junctional epithelium. Histologists think that junctional epithelium is a remnant of the enamel organ ("reduced enamel epithelium") left over as the tooth erupted. Wherever it comes from, this epithelium is unique in that it is very porous, like a membrane. It is designed to produce a constant flow of sulcular fluid; this fluid contains antibodies and even white blood cells to fight the bacteria that live in the mouth. The fluid also helps to keep the marginal gingiva in position flat against the tooth even in the absence of saliva; like a flat, thin rubber stopper in a wet sink or tub, the marginal gingiva is meant to form a tight seal against the tooth with the moisture between them.

None of the epithelium of the mouth is as keratinized as skin is, so it can be subject to trauma during activities like chewing. However, the periodontium and oral mucosa are highly vascularized, and the generous circulation of blood through the tissues aids in rapid healing. The attached gingiva has such a profuse blood supply that it is almost impossible to incise it in such a way that the blood supply is compromised. The blood supply of the oral mucosa in the antrum and the vestibule of the mouth (the free space between lips or cheeks and the teeth/periodontium) is generally at right angles to the attached gingiva. The surface of the roof of the mouth, called the palatal mucosa, functions like attached gingiva because it is firmly adhered to the palatal bone. In the caudal part of the mouth, it continues without bone as the soft palate, an arch of connective tissue covered by epithelium that separates the caudal part

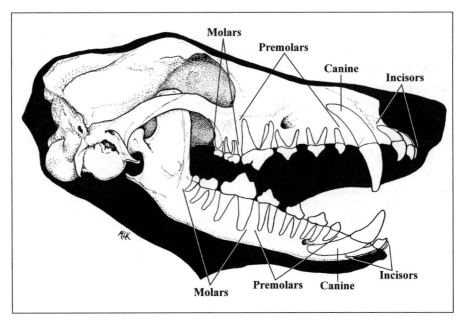

Figure 1-8

The skull of the dog showing the position and number of teeth and their roots.

of the nasal cavity from the oral cavity. The palatal mucosa is served by palatal arteries that run rostrally (forward, or toward the front) adjacent to the teeth after perforating the palatal bone medial to the upper fourth premolar. The palatal mucosa is thrown up into folds, called rugae (a single one is a ruga), which apparently aid in swallowing.

An area sometimes mentioned in stomatitis in cats, as well as some other conditions, is the fauces. This is the mucosa-covered area caudal to the back teeth and soft palate that forms the arch just rostral to the pharynx.

MORE INFORMATION ON NORMAL ANATOMY AND TERMINOLOGY

All veterinary dental texts contain dental formulas for dogs and cats. The dental formula for the mature dog is I3/3, C1/1, P4/4, M2/3 (Fig. 1-8). This translates as saying that for each side of the mouth the dog has three incisors in the front of the top jaw (the maxilla) over three incisors in the bottom jaw (the mandible), followed by one canine top and bottom, followed by four premolars top and bottom, followed by two molars over three, for a total of 42 when you count both sides. The formula for an immature animal uses lowercase letters for deciduous teeth. The formula for the puppy is i3/3, c1/1, p3/3, for a

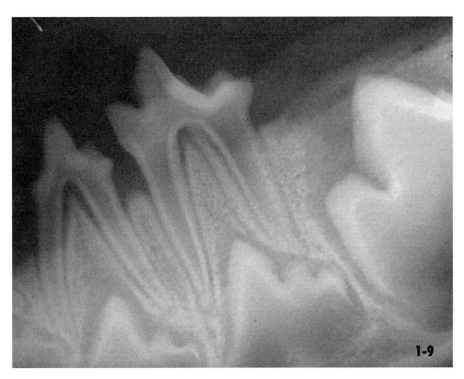

Figure 1-9

A radiograph of a puppy of about 12 weeks. The crowns of the permanent teeth are forming under the deciduous teeth. The first molar crown (right) does not have a deciduous precursor.

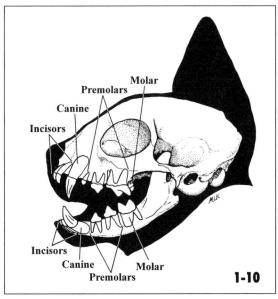

Figure 1-10

The skull of the cat showing the position and number of teeth and their roots.

total of 28 (Fig. 1-9). The formula for the adult cat is I3/3, C1/1, P3/2, M1/1 (total 30) (Fig. 1-10). The kitten formula is i3/3, c1/1, p3/2 (total 26). In actual fact the formula does not tell you much unless you can identify the teeth for what they are by form and function.

The incisors are easy to recognize because they are the front teeth and generally are the same shape. They are single-rooted teeth with short crowns and relatively long roots. Their purpose is fine gnawing, as for chewing meat off of a bone or grooming (biting an itch). The crowns of the upper incisors have a small shelf on their caudal edge, called a cingulum (plural, cingula), on which tips of the lower incisors rest when the mouth is closed in a "normal" scissors-type bite. ("Bite" here means the way the teeth fit together.) In the scissors bite, which is a term generally referring to the relationships of the incisors and canines, the upper incisors fit closely over the lower incisors to effect a shearing action. Also, the canines come together in such a way that the lower canine fits between the upper third incisor and the lower canine, equidistant and near but not touching these two teeth. Breeding of domestic dogs (and cats) has led to alterations in the normal or wild-type bite. Many breed associations accept a level (tip to tip) bite or one in which mandibular incisors are far rostral to the maxillary incisors (e.g., the "underbite" of the boxer).

The function of the canines is to grasp prey and tear flesh. The single roots on these massive teeth are slightly longer than the crowns. Since the lower canine is rostral to the upper, there is more room for an additional tooth (third molar) in the caudal mandible of dogs (cats, with their shorter jaws, have only one molar).

The premolars of dogs and cats are useful for mastication (chewing) of meat. They have pointed, triangle-shaped crowns for that purpose. However, they vary widely in their shape and size and have from one to three roots. The terminology for animal teeth comes from the human model, in which all the teeth except the molars have deciduous precursors and in which the premolars ("bicuspids") are all very much alike. In dogs, the first premolar does not have a deciduous precursor (it is permanent only, like the molar) and is a single-rooted, simple tooth. Cats lack the first premolar in the maxilla, and the first and second premolars in the mandible. Plus, there is another confusing factor about the deciduous lower fourth premolar; in the puppy or kitten it takes the shape of the first molar and interacts with the upper fourth premolar like the first molar will when it erupts! This has led some authors to assert that puppies and kittens have a lower first molar, when in fact the tooth is a premolar because its secondary tooth bud develops into a fourth premolar.

The reason that this deciduous tooth takes the shape of a molar is because of the importance of the occlusion of the upper fourth premolar and lower first molar (permanent teeth). These two teeth are called the carnassial (meaning meat-eating) teeth. They are the largest and most massively rooted of the caudal teeth, and the young animal needs the function of these teeth just as the mature animal does. Like the incisors, these teeth pass close to each other to shear through meat or other tough substances. The upper carnassial is designed to pass lateral to the lower as it does this.

In a mature dog or cat, the proper way to assess which tooth you are looking at is to identify the carnassials and count down as you go forward; if there is a premolar missing, there is generally a small gap, and if there is a duplicate of a premolar (a supernumerary tooth), it will generally be crowded. (Note: Any tooth may appear as a supernumerary tooth, as a complete extra tooth, or as a malformed part of a tooth.)

The ideal orientation for the premolars of dogs is for the tip of the crown of one to point between the teeth of the opposite jaw, although this orientation is seldom exactly perfect.

Molars are designated as grinding teeth; as such they have relatively flat, wide surfaces to grind up tough vegetable material. This is true of the dog, which naturally eats almost anything presented to it (the dog is an omnivore), but the cat is a true carnivore, as shown by its teeth, which are all sharp and pointed. The cat's two molars include (1) the tiny, almost hidden one caudal to the upper fourth premolar and (2) the lower carnassial tooth. One feature of molars as seen in dogs is that they show "cusps," the mounds on the chewing (occlusal) surfaces that roughly correlate to the roots below.

The only tooth that normally has three roots in a cat is the upper fourth premolar (although the upper third and the molar may occasionally present with three). In the dog, the upper fourth premolar and the two molars caudal to it have three roots, although the roots of the second molar are very short. It is important to know the number of roots a tooth has because multiple-rooted teeth usually need to be sectioned to remove each root separately. The area between the roots is called the furcation. It is normally filled with bone but may lose the bony attachment with periodontal disease. Teeth in the mandible never have more than two roots.

We have so far identified teeth by type and number as counted from the center of the front backward. This is called anatomic nomenclature (Figs. 1-11 and 1-12). Each tooth can be designated by a letter with a number as a superscript or a subscript; which side of the letter the number is on indicates the side of the head, and whether it is a superscript or a subscript indicates whether it is upper or lower.

Many people prefer to use a system of nomenclature called the Modified Triadan System, in which each tooth has a number (Figs. 1-11 and 1-12). The teeth are assigned a number starting with "1" from the midline around the dental arch, with each quadrant of the mouth being assigned a hundred digit to be placed in front of the tooth number, 1 for the upper right, 2 for the upper left, 3 for the lower left, and 4 for the lower right. Thus the upper right third incisor is tooth 103, the upper left fourth premolar is 208, the lower left first molar is 309, and so on. Systems of dental nomenclature are important

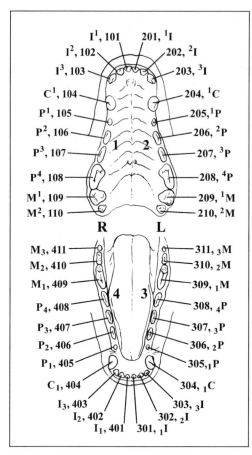

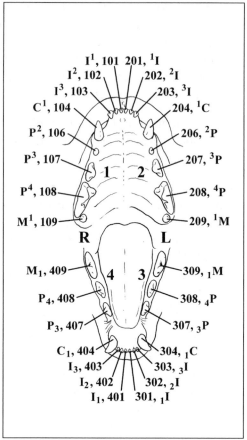

Figure 1-11

An open-mouth view of the dog with teeth identified by the anatomic and Modified Triadan System of nomenclature.

Figure 1-12

An open-mouth view of the cat with teeth identified by the anatomic and Modified Triadan System of nomenclature.

for exactly identifying teeth for oral communication and charting the teeth. The Modified Triadan System at first seems awkward but is actually an efficient shorthand.

Some other terms that will prove useful, if not essential, include descriptive terms for directions. As you move around the dental arch from the midline, you are moving in a distal direction; the surface of the tooth that is facing away from the midline is the distal surface (Fig. 1-13). The surface of the tooth toward the midline as you travel around the arch is the mesial surface or face of the tooth, and you can speak of moving in a mesial direction. The surface of the tooth facing the lips is labial; farther back in the mouth, caudal

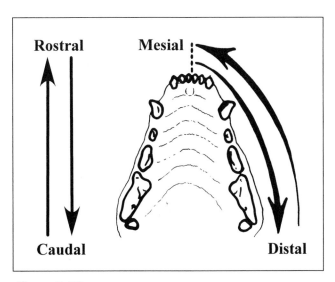

Figure 1-13

The maxillary teeth of a cat show the directions mesial and distal. On any given tooth, the mesial surface is the side nearest the middle of the incisors as you follow the arcade of the teeth; the distal surface is the side away from the midline. Note that only in the cheek teeth do the terms mesial and distal correspond to the terms rostral and caudal. The occlusal surfaces of the teeth are those that meet each other (or food during chewing).

to the commissure of the lips, the surface facing outward is called buccal because it is facing the cheek. To the inside of the mouth the surface is called either palatal (upper arcade) or lingual (lower arcade). The surfaces or edges of the tooth crowns that contact each other and food during chewing are the occlusal surfaces. The area between adjacent crowns along the arcade is called the interproximal space. If you are talking about a direction in a particular tooth root, *apically* means "toward the tip of the root," and *coronally* "toward the crown." *Cervically* ("toward the neck, or cervical region, of the tooth," which is at the cemento-enamel junction) and *occlusally* can be used to describe directions on the crown as well as *mesially* and *distally*. Studying Figures 1-11, 1-12, and 1-13 should help this terminology make sense.

We have covered a tremendous quantity of material about teeth and associated structures in this chapter. For those unfamiliar with dental terminology and structure, it will be a challenge to try to assimilate all of this factual information. However, there are two important points that should be understood by every student:

Teeth and associated structures are live tissues (with the exception of enamel) that function according to general laws of physics and physiology, as do similar tissues of the rest of the body. As living tissues they are constantly developing, maturing, maintaining, or repairing themselves; they are part of a dynamic system.

An understanding of the anatomy and physiology of teeth and periodontal tissues, and a mastery of elementary terminology pertaining to them, make up the foundation for becoming a veterinary dental technician.

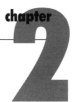

Maintaining Dental Equipment and Supplies

The dental technician is virtually always responsible for keeping inventory, ordering, cleaning, organizing, and repairing (or arranging for repairs) of all dental equipment and supplies. Without these critical services the dental operatory would grind to a standstill because dental work is so reliant on equipment.

BASIC EQUIPMENT FOR THE DENTAL OPERATORY

As a minimum, the dental operatory needs a table, hand instruments, and a polisher for dental prophies. However, even in practices that do not specialize in small animal dentistry, simple prophies are only a part of the dental caseload—extractions, oral mass removals, periodontal treatments, and simple endodontics (pulp caps) require equipment as well.

Large Equipment

For a basic setup, the table is ideally a flow table that can carry away the sometimes copious amounts of water and blood that can result from periodontal treatments and extractions (Fig. 2-1). It need not be exclusively dedicated to dentistry; many "dirty" procedures, such as cleaning out abscesses, can be done at the dentistry table. The table needs to be at a working height, since even a few hours bent over a table that is too low will result in debilitating back pain. The table should be between elbow and shoulder height when the technician is seated to do the prophy. The chair or stool height should be adjustable for different sizes of people so that they can maintain good posture while cleaning teeth (keeping the back straight and working

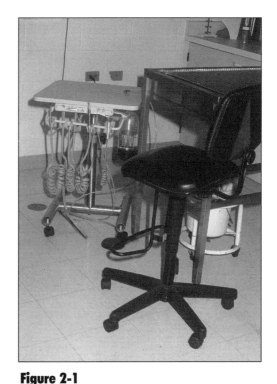

Figure 2-1
A flow table and large equipment in a dental operatory.

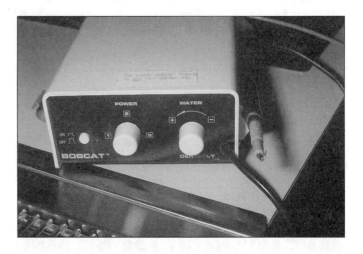

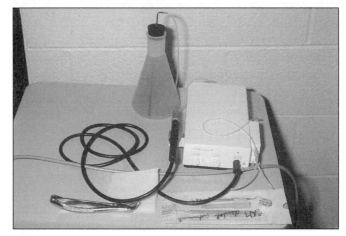

Figure 2-2

Ultrasonic scalers. The handpiece is operated by a foot pedal or a switch on the handpiece, and a water supply for cooling comes from the sink plumbing or a reservoir.

from the shoulder, not the wrist!). A solid table can be used for dental procedures but must be supplemented with adequate towels to absorb all of the generated liquid.

An ultrasonic scaler (Fig. 2-2) is virtually a necessity for any practice that performs more than one prophy in a day—in essence, all practices! The reason for this is not that the ultrasonic scaler is better but because it is much faster, particularly on thin, widespread calculus. The oscillation of the head of the ultrasonic scaler knocks the calculus off much more quickly than if the entire surface had to be scraped by hand. Several brands of ultrasonic scalers are available. Most oscillate in a forward-and-back motion at the tip, but some describe an oval or round pattern. Those with a more complicated movement are usually much more expensive but not necessarily more efficacious. The more movement and power, the greater the capacity to heat up and harm the tooth. The ultrasonic scaler should have a power rating from 40,000 to

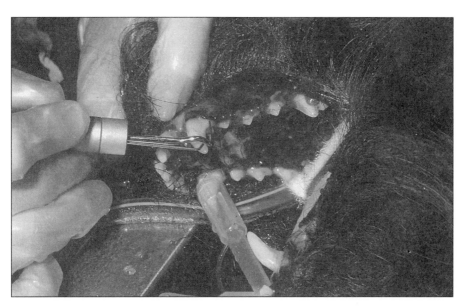

Figure 2-3
Ultrasonic scaler tips come in two general styles, either pointed or chisel edged. The pointed tip is used on its side.

100,000 hertz (cycles per second). If it has a variable power dial, it usually should be cranked to the most powerful setting in order to clean off calculus faster (which, of course, is its purpose).

Ultrasonic scaler tips generally come in two styles. One is a curved tip that tapers to a blunted point, and the other is a bent or curved tip that ends in a thin, broad edge ("chisel tip"). Remembering that the usual motion is forward and back at the tip, it is obvious that the end of the pointed tip should never be pushed directly into the tooth; this tip should be directed on its side to remove broad areas of calculus (Fig. 2-3). If it is driven into the tooth surface, it will excavate a pit, just like its large cousin the jackhammer. The chisel tip is used flat against the tooth, to push broad areas of calculus off. It is important to make sure, when installing a new chisel tip, that the edges are rounded, not sharp. Sharp edges will damage the enamel by pounding microscopic lines into it.

There are also "sonic" scalers and rotating metal burs available, but the sonic scalers are not very powerful, and the metal burs can cause severe damage to the enamel if used incorrectly (i.e., anything beyond a very light touch) and are not recommended.

The microscopic damage that the ultrasonic or any other power scaler imparts, even when used correctly, *must* be smoothed off with a polisher.

Mechanical polishers can be purchased for a few hundred dollars. They work by use of a motor and rotating shaft, which can be subject to binding. If a dental air unit is purchased for a drill, it can run a polisher as well. Air-driven polishers require a slow-speed handpiece and a prophy angle for the polishing cup. Rubber polishing cups are either snap-on or have a brass insert imbedded into them to screw into the prophy angles, which are available in snap-on, screw-on, or latch-on shaft styles. Occasionally a mechanical or an air-driven unit will fail in the middle of a procedure. For this situation, the easiest and quickest solution is to have available a battery-powered polisher, which can be purchased in human pharmacies in the dental care products section. Rubbing polish over the teeth by hand with gauze is a very poor second choice.

The dental air unit (Fig. 2-4) is a sort of symbol (along with the dental X-ray unit) of a complete dental service because of its high-speed dental drill. There are mechanical drills available, but they are very expensive and do not include water-coolant capacity. The dental drill has water supplied to the handpiece to cool the bur as it enters tooth or bone. The air unit also has, in addition to the slow-speed polisher, the air/water syringe. This convenient device provides air for drying or a water spray, or a combination of the two. The combination readily zips the teeth clean and washes away debris so that further work is possible. The air unit has a water reservoir or the capability of tapping into the office water supply. Reservoirs are adequate if they are large enough to last for a day's work and need not be refilled midway, which requires turning off the air source. It should be noted that the reservoir may potentially be contaminated with microbes.

The source of "air" for these units is actual air (via compressor), bottled carbon dioxide or nitrogen, or a hand-pump on the unit that pressurizes the reservoir. The hand-pumping unit is not recommended because each "pumping" lasts only a short time and is disruptive to the flow of the work. Large bottles of inert gas can provide power, but it is necessary to keep one in reserve for when the active bottle runs out. Nitrogen is superior to carbon dioxide because the carbon dioxide seems to have more of a tendency to freeze at the valve as it is utilized. Neither one should cause any problems in a well-ventilated hospital in the amounts released by a dental unit. Of course, too much of either gas, with the elimination of oxygen, is the foundation of a method of euthanasia for laboratory animals. The dental unit should never be attached to oxygen because sparks created by the drill could cause a flash fire. Air from a compressor eliminates the bother of gas bottles, but it creates another problem—noise. If the compressor is to be in the same room as the procedure, it must be one of the special "silent" compressors, which cost a great deal more than a standard commercial compressor. These silent compressors are also of small capacity, designed for one air unit, and may be more

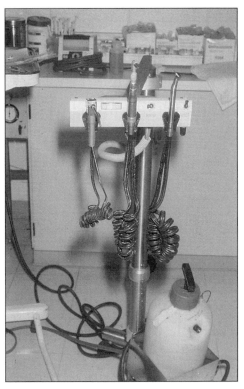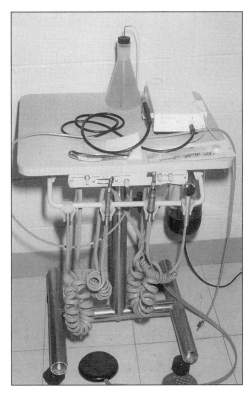

Figure 2-4
Two types of dental air unit. Notice foot pedals and reservoirs for water.

subject to breakdown with hard use. A better answer is to have the compressor and reservoir air tank in another room with a sound barrier.

Maintenance of Large Equipment

A practice that has a dental operatory and dental equipment should have a working relationship with a dental equipment maintenance/repair service. This type of business may be found in multiple listings in the yellow pages of large metropolitan areas but is not typically available locally in other areas. However, most places, even smaller towns, have one or more dentists (for human patients) who utilize equipment similar to the veterinary dentist's. These other dentists must have their equipment serviced; many are quite approachable and will tell you the service providers with whom they do business. A travel charge from a distant center might be shared if you coordinated regular service visits with one or more dentists. Probably, with the volume of dental patients most veterinarians have, a semiannual or annual maintenance visit will be adequate to keep equipment functioning. Then, when something critical breaks down unexpectedly, the service already knows you as a regular customer and is more likely to put you high on the list for a visit.

Service personnel can also help you with questions on how to use items that you might have inherited and that are a mystery to you, such as the slow-speed handpiece you cannot figure out how to install or to remove a prophy head from. They will have seen or worked on a large variety of brands and will be a valuable resource for you, especially when your dental operatory is new. There is nothing like an expert to get a system really functioning efficiently.

The best thing that a technician can do is to save the manufacturer's instructions (see below) and follow them religiously. If, however, your equipment was purchased secondhand, or if instructions were lost, or if you only rarely use the air unit, the following are some general guidelines for caring for equipment.

The first consideration is the power that supplies the air unit—the compressor. Most compressors have a valve that allows the release of the water produced from "squeezing" the air into the storage unit, the air tank. Water is accumulated in the tank faster in a humid climate than in a dry climate. If it is not drained periodically, it will affect the efficiency of the compressor and cause the tank to rust. To drain the tank, the compressor must be off, and all the pressure released. The valve is on the bottom of the tank. It is usually a butterfly knob that is turned until water flows, then tightened before the compressor is started up again. The accumulation of more than a few drops of water means that you are not draining the tank often enough. If the compressor also requires lubrication, there are usually some instructions on the equipment. Compressors (especially large, quiet ones) can be quite costly and should be well maintained. One thing that affects maintenance is continuous use. If multiple drills/polishers are on the same air source, or if use of one unit has been nearly continuous, it is worth checking the compressor occasionally. Leaks in the lines can also cause excessive activity of the compressor. An overextended compressor can overheat and "seize" like a car engine. In most practices, the compressor is turned off at night for safety.

The air unit works on a simple principle of pressurized air pushing an air turbine (like a windmill) inside the handpieces and, when the water valve is opened, pushing water out of the reservoir. The slow- and high-speed handpieces (Figs. 2-5 and 2-6) differ only in the gears in the handpiece, like the gears of a bicycle. Each volume of air, like each turn of the bicycle's pedals, makes the wheels turn more or fewer times (high or low speed) according to the gears. However, one thing to remember with an air turbine, as opposed to a bicyclist's legs, is that air doesn't have much "muscle" behind it. That is why an air drill, when it is spinning at over 100,000 rpm (revolutions per

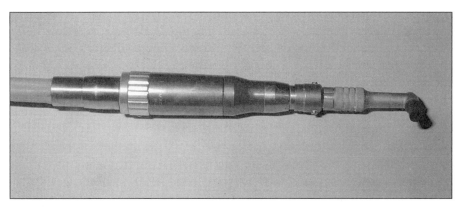

Figure 2-5
The slow-speed handpiece with prophy (polishing) angle. The handpiece should be on a regular schedule of cleaning to avoid poor performance due to gunk.

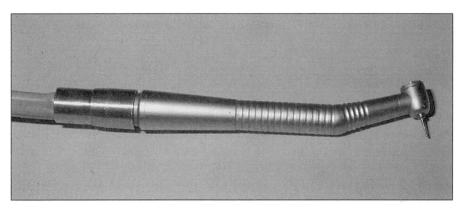

Figure 2-6
The high-speed handpiece for the dental drill. Regular oiling will ensure smooth operation and decreased wear of working parts.

minute) and making the high-pitched whining sound that puts your teeth on edge until you get used to it, dramatically drops in sound pitch when it is applied to a tooth (and may even stop revolving if pushed too hard against it) or when the prophy head's gears are too dirty and fouled with gunk to turn efficiently.

Regular maintenance of high- and low-speed handpieces is the responsibility of the technician. The metal parts of the handpieces need lubrication to run smoothly and to avoid unnecessary wear (unless they are the special handpieces that require no lubrication). All handpieces are best maintained by following the recommendations on the inserts, which also give information on, for example, how to put handpieces together and troubleshoot problems. The intervals between lubrications vary according to use; because most veterinary practices utilize handpieces less frequently than a human dentist's office does, their handpieces may need less frequent lubrication. However, it is best to follow the manufacturer's recommendations until you are completely confident with the equipment. Dirty, sludgy gears are a sign that maintenance is not thorough or frequent enough.

Slow-speed handpieces, those that are used to drive the prophy heads that carry prophy cups that polish teeth, are usually more frequently used than high-speed handpieces. Inside slow-speed handpieces there are gears that cause the air rushing through under pressure to turn the instrument at fewer revolutions per minute than high-speed handpieces. They usually vary from a 5,000 to 25,000 rpm maximum. As with the high-speed handpiece, the amount of air released through the foot pedal can vary the speed from zero to the maximum according to foot pressure (like a car's accelerator) and the resistance at the working end of the instrument.

The handpiece is attached to the air supply with a plastic coupler that accepts tubes from the handpiece. Four-hole couplers are fairly standard, but there are other configurations. It is always important to attend to which is the lubricating hole (the smaller of the larger tubes). Usually only a couple of drops are needed in the lubricating hole—the extra oil is blown out. High-speed handpieces can be stored with the heads downward to facilitate the oil getting into the working parts. Fine machine oil should be used to lubricate dental handpieces and heads. Handpieces come with a supply of oil when new, which often lasts for months or years at a drop or two at a time. Many manufacturers will caution not to use any but their own oil, but any oil from a dental supply house meant for this purpose will be fine.

The gears in the prophy head should be kept clean and lubricated. Most prophy heads come with a small wrench that will remove the retaining ring, which unscrews counterclockwise. Then there is a tiny rubber O ring that helps keep debris out of the gears. The gear that attaches to the prophy cup can be lifted out of the face of the prophy head and cleaned. The teeth of the main gear within the shaft of the prophy head can be picked out with a sharp instrument and cotton-tipped applicator. Alcohol seems to be a good solvent, and it is a mild disinfectant as well. Alcohol should be thoroughly dried (it does this spontaneously) and the parts lightly oiled before reassembly. It should be obvious that no shreds of cotton or other fibers should be allowed to stay in the gears after cleaning. Ultrasonic cleaners are excellent for cleaning prophy heads. For best results, the heads should be disassembled for cleaning.

Cleanliness in dental instruments is more of an issue for humans than animals. Once the threat of HIV virus and AIDS transmission from dental instruments became known, dentists had to provide assurances to the public that patients would not be infected in their practices. There were enormous expenditures in human dental practices for autoclavable prophy heads because it was proven that not only could the heads harbor organic debris with bacterial contaminants but also intact red and white blood cells and viable viruses. If every animal dental patient gets a new or disinfected rubber prophy cup, there is probably little reason to provide them with an autoclaved prophy head as well because it is so unlikely that they will be in contact with the organic debris that might lie within the prophy head. But certainly the equipment should be surface clean and disinfected between patients.

Mechanical parts can always wear out, so a spare prophy angle and contra angle (for the high-speed drill) are always a good idea. Gear teeth in prophy angles wear out or break off, rendering them useless. Contra angles may have chuck problems (the bur won't stay tight) or turbine problems; if you are very clever, you can replace these (most people simply discard them, however). It might be worth keeping items you consider broken to have your service person evaluate them and possibly get them reconditioned.

There are some high-speed handpieces that have fiber-optic lights. The light-bulbs are in the handpiece and are fairly easy to change.

▶ *The Reference Notebook*

The instructions for use and repair of all major dental equipment and parts, as well as all supplies, should be kept in one central place. It is simply too easy to lose the directions on how to insert and lock a drill or prophy head onto a handpiece if they are kept in the box that the handpiece came in. Or step-by-step instructions for a seldom-used cement can be accidentally dis-carded if they are left out of the box. One way to keep instructions is to dedicate a loose-leaf notebook to this purpose (or two notebooks, one for equipment and one for supplies) (Fig. 2-7). The notebook is filled with clear plastic sleeves in which the information is kept. The clear plastic not only allows both sides of a sheet to be read without taking it out but also protects the sheet from the moisture and debris that often accompany dental activities. Most of the protective plastic sleeves are double layers folded back on themselves, and not full pockets, so it might be necessary to tape instructions in place to keep them from sliding out of the sleeve. This is especially pertinent when instructions are less than a full-sized sheet. Another thing that will often help is to enlarge instructions on a copier so that the text is easier to read (many of these instructions are printed in very small type to fit the entire text on a small insert in a box). Finally, it is worthwhile to use a highlighter for the most important words in the instructions so that (for instance) you do not have to read all product endorsements or skip through French or German versions before finding the step-by-step instructions you will want to refer to again and again.

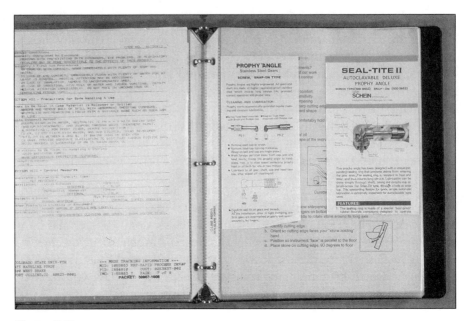

Figure 2-7

A loose-leaf notebook may be used for easy reference to, for example, maintenance of equipment and materials mixing directions.

What should be included in this notebook besides product inserts? This notebook would be a good place to list products by location (e.g., "refrigerator"), date of purchase, vendor (with address or telephone—it is very annoying, when something needs to be replaced, to have to search through numerous catalogs to find it), and cost (for cost accounting). When equipment is discarded, the information in the notebook should be discarded or entries deleted also. If equipment is replaced, it is not necessary to substitute the same insert with a newer piece of paper containing the same information nor is it necessary to have one or more duplicate inserts because, for instance, you have two of the same high-speed handpieces.

Even if all staff members are well acquainted with how to use and maintain present equipment and supplies, it is still prudent to have such a notebook. When staff changes, as it inevitably does, the notebook can serve as a valuable instructional book for new people.

Hand Instruments

The hand instruments are the backbone of the prophy. As already mentioned, the prophy can be performed with hand instruments alone, but they are more efficiently employed as clean-up tools after using the ultrasonic scaler (see Chap. 5).

For the prophy, the main instruments that are utilized are scalers and curettes, plus a dental calculus forceps or extraction forceps to crack thick calculus off the teeth before scaling, and a periodontal probe. Dental scalers may look very similar to curettes in shape but are distinguished by sharpness at the point and the cross section of the working blade. Scalers come to a sharp point at the tip and have a triangular cross section (much like a "cutting" surgical needle). Curettes have a rounded point and a **D**-shaped cross section. The reason for this is that only curettes, with their rounded edges (which are less likely to damage soft gingival attachments), are to be used subgingivally. The sharp points of the scalers can be utilized to dig calculus out of the fissures of the crowns of the teeth.

The dental hygienist who cleans your teeth has a variety of scalers and curettes for performing the prophy. These scalers and curettes come in an almost infinite variety (at least, the numbers in a catalog can make your head swim). Part of the reason that there is so much variety is that some shapes and angulations, for instance, are designed to be used only on one face of one tooth. The hygienist has the disadvantage of sitting next to you with little ability to adjust your head or twist your neck slightly while working. As a veterinary technician, you have a lot of latitude with your anesthetized patient and therefore do not need as many specialized tools. You can get by with a greatly reduced number of instruments. The majority of the prophy on many animals is performed with the ultrasonic scaler, so a single curette and a periodontal probe may be all that you will need.

As a general rule, purchasing dental instruments is like purchasing surgical instruments. The instruments with better (harder) metal and more delicate and precise working ends are more expensive. They are worth the cost because of the convenience of staying sharp longer. However, it is not the best idea to buy the high end of dental instruments on the first purchase. Rather, buy moderately expensive items, find out what you like, and then slowly build up your equipment. We autoclave or gas sterilize (because of plastic/rubber handles) a curette and a periodontal probe for each prophy. The rest of the hand equipment, which is not used on each prophy (elevators, extraction forceps, needleholders, scissors, etc.), is kept in a cold sterilization tray. Each hospital must find its own system, but the limiting factor must be that equipment is sterilized adequately before it is used in another animal's mouth, so you must have enough equipment to allow for sterilization time.

Storing Hand Instruments

There are a variety of ways to store dental instruments after cleaning them. Many dental instruments need not be sterile, but they must be disinfected and clean, like table utensils we use for eating. Dry storage after cleaning with a disinfecting soap or detergent is adequate. One way to accomplish this is to put all used instruments in a soaking solution containing a disinfectant such as chlorhexidine and then to complete washing them at the end of the day. There are instrument holders that can be used for autoclaving or merely keeping a "set" of curettes or other hand instruments together. Another way to identify sets is to use different instrument tapes. Curettes could be one color and scalers another so that they are instantly identifiable.

Since dental instruments are sharp and capable of inflicting a wound if carelessly handled, they are best stored with protective vinyl tips on their working ends. These tips are available to fit curettes, scalers, excavators, elevators, and other instruments. They are well worth the few cents they cost, since they protect instruments from dulling due to banging against one another in a drawer or container and they protect personnel from accidental punctures. Separation of instruments into plastic trays by type (which can be labeled to make identification even quicker) will make the dental operatory more efficient. There are relatively expensive furnishings, stacks of shallow drawers on rollers, which are made for storage of dental instruments and are very handy, but regular drawer space can also be made useful with dividers.

Sharpening Hand Instruments

Sharpness determines the usefulness of the entire range of hand instruments, including scalers, curettes, and elevators. The first principle involved in sharpening every one, whether it has an angle edge (scissors, scalers, and curettes) or a knife edge (elevator), is the same. The instrument contacts the sharpening stone on the point or edge first. Otherwise, fine curls of metal will accumulate at the cutting edge, blunting it (Fig. 2-8).

The next principle is that the angle between the stone and the instrument must not change during the stroke (Fig. 2-9). Wobbling or wavering in the sharpening stroke results in rounding the edge. An untutored person can quickly dull an instrument while trying to sharpen it and can actually damage the edge so much that the instrument is rendered unusable because too much metal would have to be taken off in order to sharpen it again.

The third principle is that you use the finest (refers to the size of the grit) stone available. Stones that are labeled "fine" or are Arkansas stone are what you want. The more expensive stones may have nicely rounded edges, which can be used to clean up the inside curve of an elevator, curette, or scaler (there are also round stones available, but they break easily when dropped). However, the vast majority of sharpening that you will perform will be with a flat edge.

The fewer strokes that you can use to sharpen the edge, the better. Even the fine stones are actually taking metal away, and there is a limited amount of metal available in the working point of a delicate curette. When using a fine

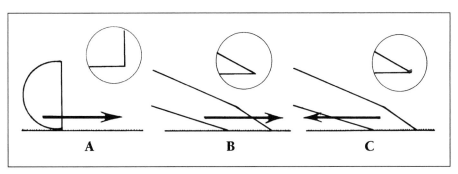

Figure 2-8
When sharpening, the edge that should be sharp always passes forward relative to
the stone, whether the instrument is like a knife blade (A) or a curette (B). If the
reverse were performed, tiny curls of metal would blunt the "sharp" edge (C).

Figure 2-9
If the angle of the instrument to the stone
changes during the stroke, the "sharp" edge
will be rounded. If enough rounding is performed on a delicate curette, it will be ruined
because there is not enough metal to restore
the sharp edge.

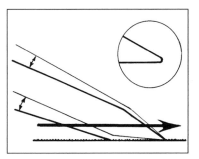

stone to sharpen, the scratches formed by the abrasion of the stone at the edge
are so tiny as to be inconsequential.

How can you tell that an instrument is dull? One way, of course, is through
feel: during use it skips and does not take calculus off, or it slips off the bone
(in the case of an elevator). Yet if we use the animal as a testing surface, we
take a contaminated instrument to the stone and contaminate the stone with
it, which would, in turn, contaminate subsequent instruments. Instruments
should be clean before sharpening to avoid carrying bacteria to the stone. (We
recommend rinsing to remove debris, then soaking used instruments in a
solution of a disinfectant such as Nolvasan for at least 20-30 minutes before
sharpening, and then gas sterilization. Preferably, clean or sterilized instruments could also be sharpened and stored prior to use on an animal.)

There is a tool that can be used to test instruments for sharpness before and
during sharpening. It is an acrylic rod. Years ago, before AIDS, hepatitis B and
C, and OSHA regulations, dental hygienists tested the sharpness of their
instruments on their fingernails. A sharp instrument lifted a thin curl of fingernail as it was lightly drawn across the nail, while the dull instrument

skipped over it. The acrylic rod is much the same consistency as our nails and ever so much safer. If bacteria or viruses are present, they cannot infect you if you keep the business ends of sharp instruments away from your body. The acrylic cases that some brands of syringe come in, or the syringe barrels themselves, are an alternative to the acrylic rod. If an OSHA inspector should see you testing instrument sharpness on your nail, he or she could "nail" you for an unsafe practice.

You can actually get a reasonably good idea about instrument sharpness visually. If, when light falls on the edge, it reflects the edge, it is rounded and dull. All you should see are the two intersecting walls, whether those are part of a knife point or for an angled edge. Magnification can make this more obvious.

There are essentially two methods for sharpening. In one the instrument is moved while the stone stays in one place, and in the other the stone is moved over an immobilized instrument (Fig. 2-10).

The most critical part of the sharpening process is establishing the correct angle and then keeping the exact same angle during every stroke against the stone. This can be done with a stationary stone by holding the curette or scaler in a modified pen grip and then moving it in a pulling motion from shoulder and elbow with your wrist fixed. The pull doesn't have to be that long—the full length of the stone, for instance, would be so long that it would tend to make you wobble. Both top and bottom edges of the curette or scaler should be sharpened, and for this you must place the stone on the edge of a counter or table because one of the angles will often put the handle below the surface of the stone. Typically the most worked edge is the bottom of the "foot" of the instrument because it is the most useful angle to use. Curettes come in two general shapes. One is the Gracie type, which has the working end of the foot of the instrument at a 40-degree angle. Universal curettes are made so that either side may be used and are set into the handle at a 90-degree angle.

For the stationary instrument technique, the instrument is held with one hand and steadied by clamping your elbow to your side. If you are right-handed, you would usually hold the instrument with your left hand. Hold the instrument within your palm rather than in a pen grip; the edge to be sharpened should be below your hand and perpendicular to the floor (so that the inside of the curve of the curette to be sharpened faces up toward the ceiling). The stone in your other hand is stroked straight down toward the floor in short motions. Two or three strokes are all that are needed for a slightly dull instrument.

Note that the curette is supposed to have a rounded, atraumatic point to the tip. As the instrument is sharpened repeatedly, the point tends to become

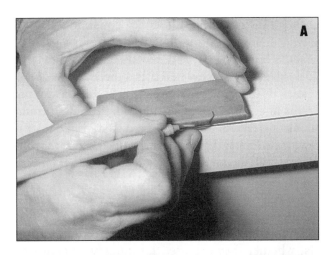

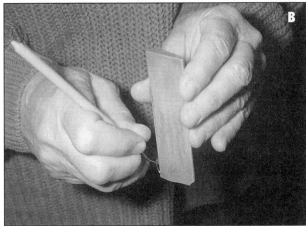

Figure 2-10

There are two general ways to sharpen instruments:

(A) the stone is kept stable on a steady surface, and the instrument is drawn over it, or

(B) the instrument is held stable in a fixed hand, and the stone is passed by it.

In both techniques, it is critical that the angle between the stone and the instrument do not waver.

sharp. The tip should be passed against the stone in a slightly rotating fashion to round it to a gentle curve.

Although there are stones advertised as "dry" stones, they are unlikely to work as well as "wet" stones. That is because the stone surface is being ground off while the metal is sharpened, and the powdery debris falls into the spaces between the grit of the stone, clogging it and rendering it useless. A fine oil is the usual wetting agent of choice for a stone. As the stone debris and the metal filings come off, they are held in suspension in the oil. If the oil gets sludgy and dark with debris, it should be wiped off, and new oil applied. Similarly, oil should not be allowed to dry on a stone when it is stored, as the debris will fill the microscopic holes in the stone. Water can be used as a wetting agent, but it does not hold the fine debris in suspension as well as oil. It could also induce rust in nonstainless steel. All oil should be wiped off the instrument before sterilization (with alcohol, if the oil is persistent). A stone that has become dirty and clogged can be washed under a stream of warm to hot water or soap and water to make it useful again.

Sterilization

A note regarding sterilization and instrument sharpness is in order. Autoclaving dulls instruments, whether they are used for surgery or dentistry, and so it results in instruments wearing out faster because they must be more frequently sharpened.

Cold sterilization and air storage are the least likely to dull stainless steel instruments. Exposure times and changes of solutions for chemical sterilants must be strictly observed to ensure complete killing of microbes. Also, instruments must look clean before being placed in the cold sterilization tray. Any organic debris (saliva, pus, blood, etc.) will inactivate the chemical sterilants. Many chemical sterilants turn cloudy with exposure to organic substances; cloudiness indicates that it's time for a change, even if the normal change interval has not passed.

Chemical sterilants are designed for stainless steel. Other metals (like that of carbide dental burs) tend to corrode and discolor the solution. Gas sterilization, if available, may be a good alternative to autoclaving or cold sterilization. One convenient way to sterilize by gas or autoclave is to use the paper packets that have a clear window on one side so that it is instantly evident what is inside.

Dental burs are difficult to get absolutely clean except by use of an ultrasonic cleaner, which some practices have for general surgical instrument cleaning. Lacking one of these, fine metal brushes are available to clean burs by hand. Autoclaving will ensure sterility and is the procedure of choice for burs. There are autoclavable holders designed to carry several burs. A stainless steel tea ball (for steeping loose tea leaves) can also be used for autoclaving and ultrasonic cleaning. Practices that do a lot of dental work will have numerous bur holders that contain commonly used burs so that a sterile bur is always available. Burs have a finite lifespan and should be discarded when dull or broken.

Dental Radiology

The technician is usually responsible for taking and developing dental X rays for the veterinarian to read. Accurate dental X rays are critical to a full-service dental practice. They aid in the diagnosis of an apical abscess or confirm the filling of a root canal. They allow the extent of the destruction of a feline resorptive lesion to be assessed and show the position of retained roots. Although there is much that can be done in dentistry through sight and touch, there are times when a diagnostic X ray is the only way to see what needs to be seen.

Today, technology is rapidly increasing the tools for veterinary dental radiology. Light, handheld X-ray units and automatic processors are becoming more common in veterinary dentistry, and digitization of images with computers may find its way into the veterinary practice. There are self-developing film packets available, which eliminate the need for bulky developing equipment of any kind. On the other hand, there are still practices that take dental radiographs with standard X-ray units.

For a moderate investment, a practice can acquire a dental X-ray unit and hand-developing chamber, which make up the present standard of care for veterinary dentistry. Dental X rays should always be taken on the small nonscreened films meant for intraoral use (Fig. 3-1). The detail obtained with these films is much finer than that achieved with screened cassettes, and they are much less expensive to use. The intraoral packets can be used with a regular diagnostic X-ray unit, but the advantage of a dental unit is its maneuverability. A fixed head X ray requires the patient to be moved into the ideal position, whereas the dental machine can be moved freely around the patient—everywhere

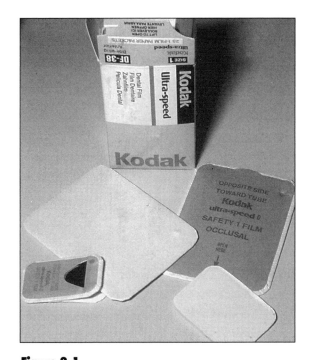

Figure 3-1
Nonscreen dental X-ray film.

except directly underneath. In addition the beam is coned very tightly in a dental machine (with little scatter radiation) to accommodate the small target.

Modern dental X-ray machines have other advantages as well. The energy used is much lower than in machines that must penetrate much thicker tissue, and on newer machines the kVp and MA are preset. This means that the time of exposure is the only variable, which makes the unit easier to use. It also means that no special shielding need be used for dental X-ray rooms and that even if the machine is aimed directly at someone (which is not a good idea!) the dose would be negligible at greater than 6 ft (approximately 2 m) distance. These modern machines are also quite inexpensive compared with the standard units and can be very useful for X rays of pocket pets and birds.

The intraoral film packets come in several sizes to fit a variety of mouths (Fig. 3-2). The smallest is size 0, which is useful for taking the tiniest of images, such as the caudal mandible of a cat. Slightly larger size 1 also fits in a cat's mouth and has a format that is longer and generally more useful. Size 2 is useful for single images of teeth or several teeth in a row on a smaller dog or for a view of the canines of the upper or lower jaw of a cat (rostral maxillary or rostral mandibular view). Size 4 is the largest of the intraoral films; it is critical for the rostral maxillary or mandibular view of larger dogs and is often used for most of the rest of the views for dogs as well because of the length of their jaws and the size of their teeth.

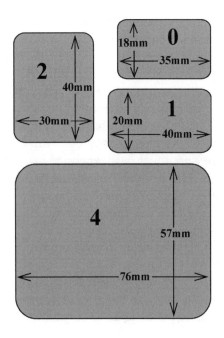

Figure 3-2

Dental X-ray film comes in four sizes, shown here. Size 2 and 4 are the most convenient in veterinary dentistry, although sizes 0 and 1 can be useful in cats and very small dogs.

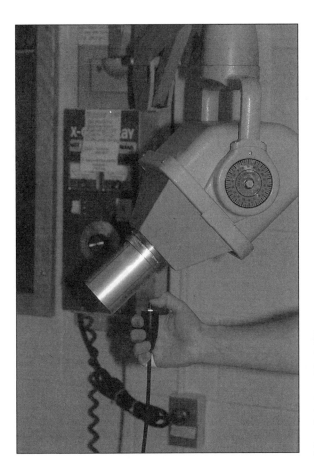

Figure 3-3
The head of the dental X-ray machine can be manipulated to almost any angle, and the expandable trigger cord allows the operator to remove him- or herself from the X-ray beam.

RADIOLOGICAL SAFETY

Safety precautions must always be observed when using any X-ray equipment. All personnel should be wearing personal dosimeters, or film badges, when working around X rays. No needless exposure of personnel should be allowed, especially of women of childbearing age. When dental X rays are shot, everyone should leave the area and preferably stand behind a wall or door and definitely out of the direct beam, regardless of how far away. In the exceptionally rare situation that someone is needed to hold an animal, all protective clothing should be worn (apron, gloves, thyroid guard), and the person should avoid being in the direct beam. More than one trigger is preferable because a fixed trigger within the room could be in the line of fire. Most machines have a coiled expandable cord trigger that will allow the operator to stand 10 or 15 ft away from the X-ray head in any position in the room, or even outside the room (Fig. 3-3).

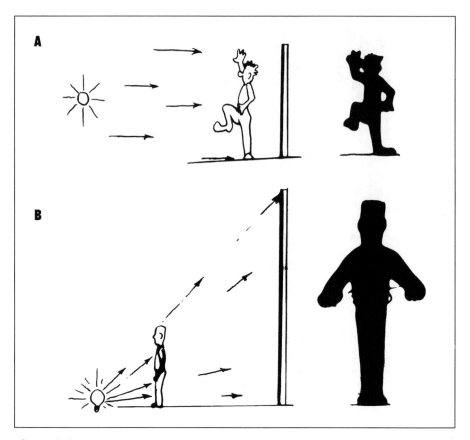

Figure 3-4

Light beams act a great deal like X-ray beams.

(A) If the light source is very far away, or if X-ray beams are trapped within a cone so that the photons of light or the X rays are nearly parallel, the "shadows" cast will be nearly the same size as the object if object and image surface are parallel to each other and perpendicular to the beam.

(B) If the light source or the X-ray source is close to the object, and relatively far from the image surface, there will be magnification of the image.

POSITIONING

The least distortion in an image occurs when the source (focal point) of X rays is as far away as possible from the object and the film is as close as possible behind the object. This can be demonstrated by the use of light (Fig. 3-4). If the source of light is far away, as with sunlight, a shadow of an object cast on a surface near and parallel to it is almost exactly the same size. Yet if the light source is extremely close to the object, and the surface farther away from it, the light rays will magnify the image's size relative to the object. That is why when a thick subject is radiographed the portion closest to the film is the smallest. This is easily seen in radiographs of the temporomandibular joint (TMJ), where the joint away from the film is noticeably larger. On the other hand, with X rays the penetrating power is rapidly lost the farther from the source the object is placed. The cone of the dental X-ray machine is meant to be placed as close as possible to the object to get optimum penetrance of the beam. The cone also deletes scatter radiation, so the X rays should be as close as possible to parallel when they strike the object.

The least distortion of the radiographic image results when film and object are parallel and exactly perpendicular to the X-ray beam. The first thing that must be understood about taking radiographs of animals' teeth is that there is only one place in the mouth in which this parallel technique can be used: the caudal mandible. In all other areas adjustments must be made with a variation of the bisecting angle technique.

Looking at a cat's or dog's mouth will reveal that, unlike humans, they have a flat palate. The human palate is domed upward, which allows dental hygienists to use a parallel, or near-parallel, technique when taking intraoral radiographs. With a flat palate, the tooth and its root(s) form virtually a right angle with the film. Also, the mandibular symphysis (the bony union that is our chin) in humans is flat from front to back, and the teeth are upright, which allows parallel intraoral views of the incisors and canines. In dogs and cats, the symphysis is long from front to back and the tooth roots extend backward. However, by adjusting the angle of the beam, an image of the proper proportions of the teeth of both upper and lower jaws can be captured.

When describing the way the image appears on film in a nonparallel technique, an analogy to the shadow of a tree in sunlight can be made (Fig. 3-5). The tree and the ground are analogous to a tooth and the film when the film cannot be held parallel to the tooth because of the palate. If the sun is directly overhead, the shadow on the ground is short and broad, and only the leafy top, and not the trunk, shows in the shadow silhouette. This is what happens if the X-ray beam is aimed at a right angle (90 degrees) to the film: the roots do not show, and only the occlusal outline of the tooth is revealed. If, however, the sun is very low in the sky, the shadow thrown by the tree becomes very long, much taller than the tree. Similarly, if the X-ray beam is aimed near 90 degrees to the tooth, the image elongates excessively, and usually the root tips will not even be on the film (and the root tip is generally the most critical part of the image) (Fig. 3-6).

To make a shadow that is exactly the height of the tree, the sun must be 45 degrees from the line of the tree. This only works if the ground is flat, however. If the tree is on a hill (similar to the angle at which a tooth might be from the film), the angle of the sun must be different to throw a shadow exactly the

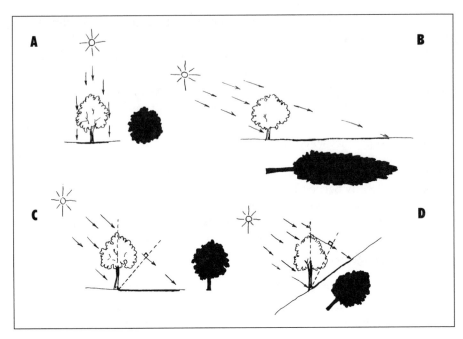

Figure 3-5

The angle of the X-ray beam, like the angle of light striking a tree and throwing a shadow, determines how accurate the height of the resulting image will be. Note what happens

(A) when the sun is overhead (as when we aim the X-ray beam at a right angle to the film and parallel to the tooth root and the image is foreshortened) or

(B) when the sun is too low (as when we aim the X-ray beam at a right angle to the tooth root and more parallel to the film) and the image elongates. Because we seldom can make dental X rays in which the tooth is parallel to the film, we must use the bisecting angle technique

(C) which is estimated by finding the plane of the film (the ground) and the axis of the tooth (the tree) and drawing a line (the bisecting angle) exactly between them. When the light is projected directly at the bisecting angle, the image on the ground is exactly the same height as the tree. If the ground is flat, the bisecting angle technique will be in effect at precisely the time the sun is halfway between sunrise and when it is directly overhead.

(D) If, however, the tree is on a hill, the bisecting angle will change, and the sun must be in a different position. When we take X rays, we must estimate the bisecting angle for each position.

height of the tree on the ground. The sun must be 90 degrees to a line drawn midway between the line of the tree and the line of the ground. This is the bisecting angle. It works exactly the same way with an X ray of a tooth, and that is the key to perfect dental radiographs (with a few variations for unique situations that are explained in the following).

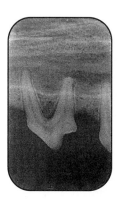 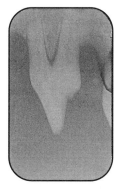

Figure 3-6

Example of two films of the same tooth. The film on the left is done with proper bisecting angle technique. The film on the right has root elongation and does not show the root apex. Some elongation can be useful, to better examine the length of the root. Foreshortened views are seldom of any use.

Figure 3-7

Survey X rays of a dog. See if you can find an anomaly (hint: count teeth). The dog's left side is on your right, and vice versa, just as if you were looking at the mouth (flattened out) from the outside.

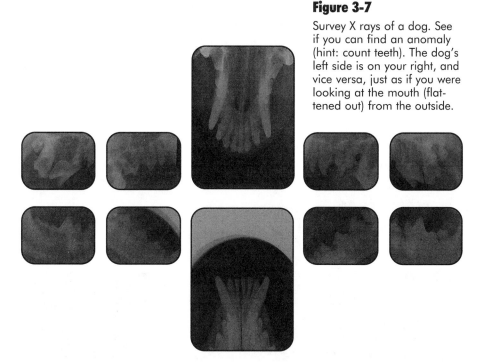

Survey radiographs are a set of X rays that show the entire mouth (Fig. 3-7). Many human dental practices routinely take survey or screening radiographs every time a patient comes in for periodic care. It is done less often in veterinary dentistry, but survey radiographs of a normal mouth can be useful for establishing a baseline and occasionally for finding a hidden abnormality, similar to screening blood work.

Survey radiographs involve at least six views for the cat (upper and lower cheek teeth on each side and both rostral upper and lower canines with incisors) (Fig. 3-8). For the dog there are at least four more views because the cheek teeth require two separate views for both upper and lower arcades as a result of the length of the jaws. In addition, it may be necessary to take more than one angle from front to back on certain multiple-rooted teeth. This is done to separate root tips that may be superimposed in a straight lateral view in both dogs and cats (how to do this is explained later).

An important step in taking a dental X ray is to place the film in the mouth in the proper position so that it will not shift if the head is moved or if there is a delay before the film is shot. In human dentistry the film packets have a cardboard flange attached to the middle of the front of the film ("bite-wing" X rays), and the patient is instructed to bite down on the flange, which holds the film firmly against the teeth inside the mouth. Our patients are anesthetized and would not hold the bite-wing packet in the mouth in 99 percent of the cases anyway, so a means of keeping the film in place must be devised.

There are several devices that aid intraoral positioning. One popular style is a sort of triangular block with a ribbed surface that allows the film packet to be

Figure 3-8

Survey X rays of a cat. This cat shows widened periodontal spaces medial to both upper canines (*see arrows*).

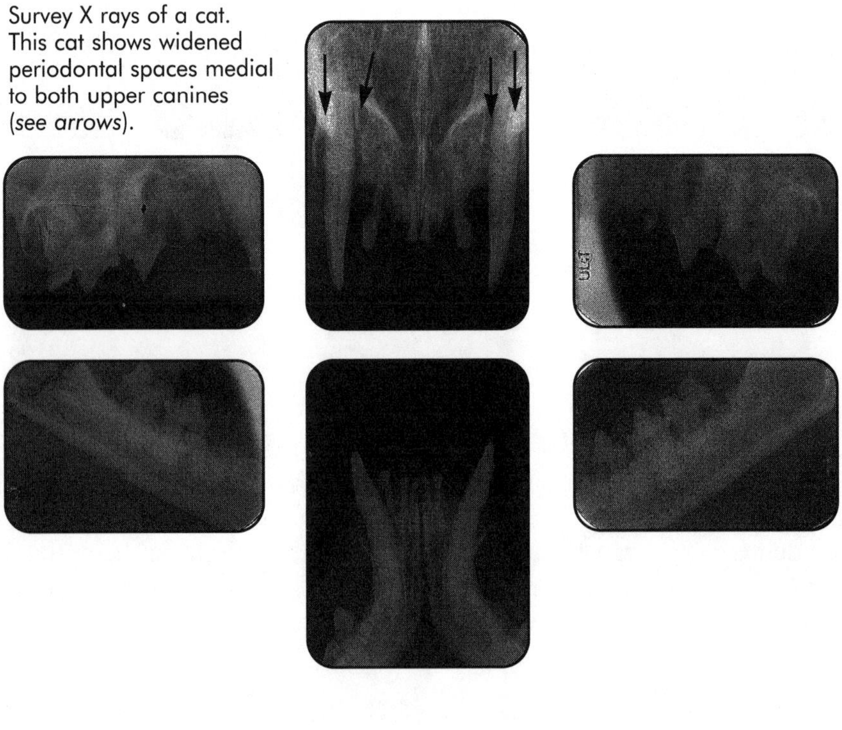

wedged in place in a variety of intraoral positions. Moldable foam curlers made for hair styling have been used to block the film packets into place. Pieces of foam rubber can be used but are impossible to clean between patients. An old standby, especially in a small mouth where a device might not fit, is wadded-up paper towels. The cheapest, least absorbent towel can be the best at holding its shape. Gauze sponges are also sometimes useful.

The only thing to avoid with all positioning aids is that the device not be between the film and the X-ray beam. Otherwise, an artifact (an image that was not cast by the tissues intended to be radiographed) may result. Regardless of the type of positioning aid, the most important thing to remember is that the proper side must face the X-ray beam; the opposite side of the packet contains lead foil, which absorbs the X rays after passing through the film and keeps them from bouncing back through the film. There will be no image on the film if the foil side is up.

A variety of pads or sandbags for positioning the head are also useful. As mentioned above, the dental X ray can be positioned virtually anywhere but under the head. However, it may be necessary to tilt the mandible up off of the table in order to shoot it from an angle slightly below parallel, for instance. If the X-ray machine has a fixed head, there is only limited angulation from straight down to the table. In this case more tortuous positioning may be necessary, even requiring holding the patient by hand (in lead-lined gloves and other protective clothing, of course).

When learning how to take dental X rays, it is a good idea to have a skull handy to look at the teeth without the confusing soft tissues (Fig. 3-9). For instance, examine how far caudal from the nose the teeth are in the average dog. The nose is a soft tissue blob that extends rostral to any incisors, except possibly in some brachycephalic animals (like bulldogs). The skull also gives indications of how superficial roots are. In particular, as you examine the maxilla, there are bulges in the bone over the roots of certain teeth. The most obvious teeth so indicated are the canine and fourth premolar. The swellings in the bone are called jugae (singular = juga). The name is not very important, but what is important is to realize that when the juga is seen, the root is only a couple of millimeters (at most) below the surface of the bone, and the line of the root can be assessed from it.

One other thing to get a feeling for before trying to take dental radiographs is the length, direction, and shape of tooth roots. A good way to begin to do this is to study a skull or, better yet, one in which the bone has been partially removed to reveal where the roots lay. If you lack this aid, a detailed dental chart or good anatomical illustrations will help. However, a single skull or illustration does not begin to show all the variations that can occur in actual animals' teeth, and nothing can replace experience and knowledge acquired

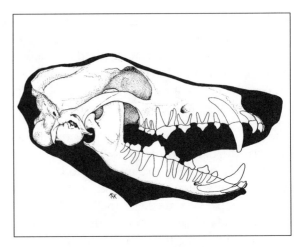

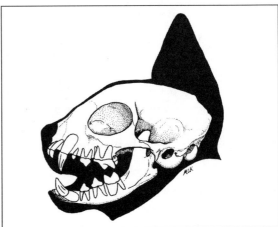

Figure 3-9

Normal dog and cat skulls. Note the positions of the roots of the teeth.

by trial and error. Everyone can expect to shoot a lot of extra radiographs while learning how to do it. In fact, shooting X rays of the clean skull for practice may speed learning the techniques.

Following are the standard views of survey radiographs and more information on the special cases mentioned above.

1. **The rostral maxillary view, dog and cat.** This is a dorsal-ventral (DV) type of view in which the X-ray beam passes from the top of the nose through the teeth and the image falls on the film. When the film is placed in the mouth, the crowns of the canines will push the front of the packet away from the palate, and although the premolars will also keep it from touching the palate, it will be

closer to the palate at the rear of the packet. In general, you always want the film to be as close to the tooth as possible, so secure the film against the canine and premolar tips. This establishes the plane of the film.

Next, the line through the canines must be established. The incisors are in another plane, so unless the incisors are the target, the canines are more important and more likely to be distorted, and their plane is the target. The apex of the canine root is almost always directly over the mesial root of the second premolar, and the tooth is curved like a banana. The plane of the tooth is approximated on this curved tooth by establishing where the tip of the crown and apex of the root are located and drawing an imaginary line through it.

Then, with the X-ray beam centered exactly over the midline of the nose, it is aimed perpendicular (90 degrees) to a line exactly midway between the plane of the film and the plane of the teeth (Fig. 3-10). It is important to have the film packet far enough back in the mouth that the image of the tip of the root falls on the film. The center of the beam should cross the center of both canine teeth.

The canines of the cat, and those of short-faced dogs, are much more upright than in a normal dog. This means that the angle between the plane of the film and that of the tooth is much more open, and the X-ray head therefore should be more in front of the face. Note that with a dental X-ray machine, this view, and all of the others, can be made with the animal on its side.

2. The rostral mandibular view, dog and cat. A similar situation exists with this ventral-dorsal (VD) view, but the roots of the canine teeth are in a flatter plane; they follow the underline of the jaw fairly closely in both species. Therefore, the beam, which is centered over the midline as before, is closer to ventral than to rostral compared with X rays of the maxilla (Fig. 3-11). It may be necessary to put a pad under the mandible to allow the beam to be fired squarely at both sides of the mandible when the animal is on its side.

3. The distal (caudal) mandibular view, dog and cat. This is the only view that can be made with a true parallel technique, as stated above (and shown in Fig. 3-12). The appropriate film is selected for

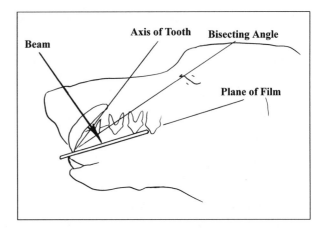

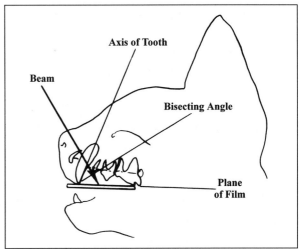

Figure 3-10

Rostral maxillary view for canines and incisors, dog and cat. Since the canine teeth are the most prominent, and usually more important, the axis of the canine tooth is used to estimate the bisecting angle with the plane of the film. The X-ray beam is pointed directly at (90 degrees to) the bisecting angle. The X-ray beam should be centered from side to side for a symmetrical view of the teeth. If only one canine is desired, the beam should be pointed at that tooth, only more from its side (in which case the view would be a rostral maxillary oblique).

the size of the animal (1 for cats and up to 4 for dogs, depending on size), and the film is placed between tongue and jaw parallel to the axis of the tooth roots to below the lower edge of the jaw. If the film will not fit that far ventrally, it may be necessary to shoot from an angle slightly ventral rather than one that is directly perpendicular to the teeth. Also, there may be an advantage in some cats of aiming from not only slightly

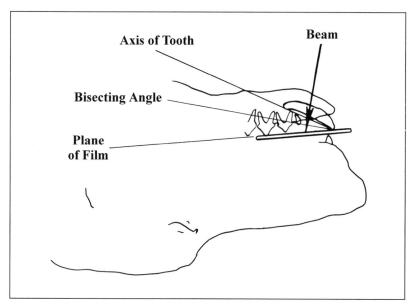

Axis of Tooth

Beam

Bisecting Angle

Plane
of Film

Figure 3-11

Rostral mandibular view for canines and incisors, dog. Again, this is a
bisecting angle technique using the axis of the canine tooth. The biggest
difficulty in this view is to push the tongue back so that it is not between
teeth and film.

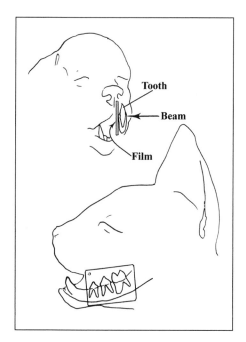

Tooth

Beam

Film

Figure 3-12

Caudal mandibular view,
dog and cat. This is the only
view of these animals that
can be done as a parallel
technique with the film
placed parallel to the teeth
and the beam pointed
directly at (90 degrees to)
both. In the cat, all the
mandibular teeth are cau-
dal to the mandibular symphysis. Some difficulty may
be met getting the film far
enough caudal because of
the soft tissue resistance,
and a firm block may have
to be used to keep the film
in place.

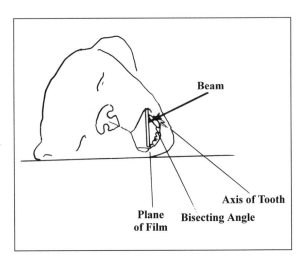

Figure 3-13

Rostral mandibular view for premolars, dog. Because the mandibular symphysis extends caudal to the second premolar in the dog, it is often necessary to do a bisecting angle technique for the roots of premolars 1 and 2.

ventral but slightly caudal as well, as the film may not fit as far back in the smaller animal's mouth. This view will get all of the mandibular premolars and molars in a cat but will be mainly a molar and fourth premolar view in a dog.

4. The rostral mandibular view for premolars, dog. The mandibular symphysis is rostral to all the mandibular cheek teeth in a cat, but in the dog the first and second premolars are rostral to it. If the film is placed in a parallel position alongside the jaw, it is forced upward by the symphysis, which can cause the roots of these first two teeth to be cut off on the X ray. To a certain extent this can be adjusted for by aiming somewhat from the ventral aspect. If this still doesn't work, a modification of the bisecting angle can be used. This is done by placing the film on the crown of the near canine and at the base of the farther canine, pushing the root of the tongue to the farther side behind the film and then aiming (from somewhat ventral) for the bisecting angle between teeth and film. This premolar view should usually overlap the caudal mandibular view to ensure all teeth and roots are seen. The beam should be aimed from the side at the middle tooth of those in the film; the ventral angle depends on accommodating the mandibular symphysis (Fig. 3-13).

5. The rostral maxillary view for premolars, dog. These rostral cheek teeth are captured on X ray with the bisecting angle technique

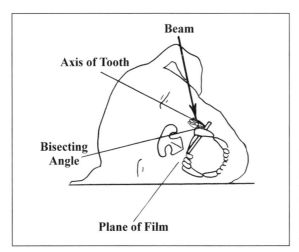

Figure 3-14
Rostral maxillary view for premolars, dog. A relatively straightforward bisecting angle technique.

(Fig. 3-14). The film is laid across the palate as close to the palate as the teeth will allow. Unless the mouth is exceptionally narrow compared with the length of the tooth roots, the film can be placed on the palate next to the opposite teeth, but it is held off the soft tissues by the crowns of the teeth to be radiographed. The beam is aimed from the side at the middle tooth in the X ray as well as from above the teeth at an angle that will be perpendicular to the line of the bisecting angle between teeth and film. This view should provide an adequate image of the one- and two-rooted first and second premolars.

6. The distal (caudal) maxillary view, dog. This is the main view of the fourth premolar and first and second molar (Fig. 3-15). Because of the flat palate, the bisecting angle technique is used as in the premolar view, with the film resting on the palate. The shot is aimed directly at the middle of the fourth premolar from about 45 degrees above the tooth. Unfortunately, this view will almost inevitably result in overlap of the mesial (rostral) roots of P4. To separate the roots (necessary, for instance, when a root canal is being performed), the X-ray head must be moved either rostrally or caudally. For most head types, the beam is shot from a more caudal position, from 30 to 45 degrees, while still aiming at P4 in a bisecting angle in the other plane. For some dolicho-cephalic heads (as in greyhounds or collies, with extremely long skulls and plenty of space between teeth) the beam is aimed at P4 from 30 to 45 degrees in front of it.

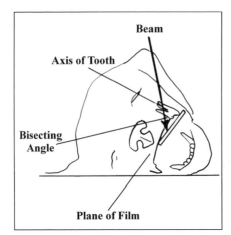
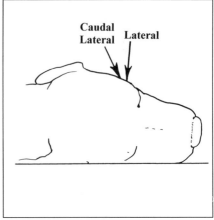

Figure 3-15

Caudal maxillary view, dog. This view is complicated by the fact that all three teeth in the caudal arch are three rooted and the line of the tooth arch curves medial in its caudal aspect. Usually the beam is aimed at a bisecting angle from directly lateral to the upper fourth premolar. This will result in overlap of the mesial buccal and palatal roots of this tooth and a somewhat occlusal view of the first and second molar. If the more caudal teeth are the targets, the beam must come from a more caudal angle, with a more correct bisecting angle for the target tooth. If there is a desire to separate the two rostral roots of the fourth premolar, the beam is moved more caudal or more rostral. The position of the roots is explained in the next figure.

Note that it is sometimes critical to separate the mesial roots of the fourth premolar and to know which is which. If two or more shots are taken, the mesial root that moves the same way as the X-ray beam is the palatal root. This is expressed by the SLOB rule: **s**ame **l**ingual (actually, palatal), **o**pposite **b**uccal. The buccal root will move the opposite direction from the beam. This means that if you take a view of the upper fourth premolar from caudal to the tooth, the root in the middle is the palatal. If you take it from rostral to the tooth, the middle root will be the mesial buccal root. You can demonstrate this phenomenon with your left hand, making the thumb the distal buccal and your first and second fingers the mesial buccal and palatal roots (Fig. 3-16).

If a view should be needed of the first or second molar specifically, the beam is moved farther caudal. These teeth are placed more medially on the palate than the upper fourth premolar and so tend to show more of an occlusal view when the carnassial tooth is well displayed.

7. The maxillary view for premolars and molar, cat. The cat's maxillary cheek teeth can be taken with one X ray, just as its mandibular cheek teeth can. However, the standard bisecting angle may not work well for the cat because the zygomatic arch is so far lateral and so

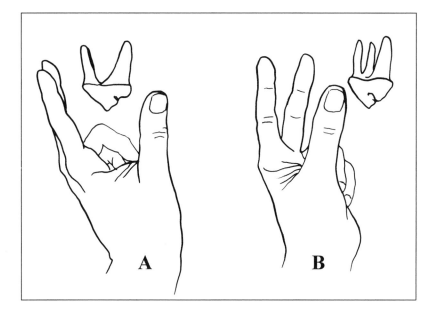

Figure 3-16

The SLOB rule. Sometimes, as with a root canal, it is necessary to know which root of the two rostral roots one is dealing with. Your eye can represent the X-ray source, and your left hand can represent the three roots of the left upper fourth premolar tooth, with the thumb as the caudal (distal) root, the index finger as the mesiobuccal root, and the middle finger as the palatal root.

(A) When your eye looks more from the index finger side, the index finger moves in front of the middle finger.

(B) When your eye looks more from the thumb side, the middle finger moves with the eye to a space between index finger and thumb. Therefore, if you move the X-ray beam caudally, the palatal root will move caudally on the film, or if you move the beam rostrally, the palatal root will move the same way. The buccal root will move the opposite direction from the direction of the head of the X-ray machine. The SLOB rule therefore stands for **s**ame (direction) = **l**ingual root (actually, palatal root, but it doesn't make as good an acronym), **o**pposite (direction) = **b**uccal root.

Figure 3-17

Maxillary view for premolars and molar, cat. Sometimes, because it sticks out so much more laterally than in the dog, the zygomatic arch of a cat will overlap the roots of the maxillary teeth, obscuring them on the X ray. One way to avoid the zygomatic arch is to lower the angle of the X ray to shoot under the bone while placing the film at a nearly parallel angle across the mouth.

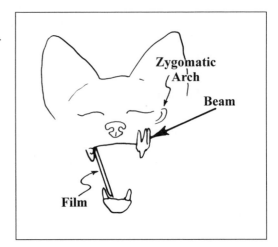

radiodense that it will obscure the roots of P3 and P4. To get these roots, a modified parallel technique is used (Fig. 3-17). So that it avoids going through the zygomatic arch, the beam is shot from a more shallow angle than for the bisecting angle technique that works so well for the dog. The film may be placed either inside or outside the mouth approximately parallel with the tooth roots. The mouth has to be propped wide open for either of these techniques. The tongue is almost always seen on the film, but it is only a soft tissue density and seldom causes confusion. If the film is placed outside of the mouth the crowns of the opposite maxillary teeth tend to intrude into the film. The mandibular crowns of either or both sides may also show on this view, especially if the mouth is not opened far enough.

8. The rostral oblique view of a canine tooth. Sometimes the second premolar overlaps the apex of the upper canine in the rostral mandibular view. If visualization of the apex is important (and it usually is!), an oblique shot of the individual canine may be required. Shooting from the same bisecting angle above the tooth that was used for the rostral mandibular view, the X-ray head is merely moved from midline to the side about 30 degrees. This will project the canine root away from the premolars.

9. The temporomandibular joint (Figs. 3-18 and 3-19).

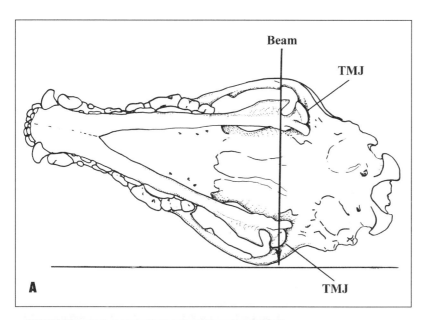

Beam

TMJ

TMJ

A

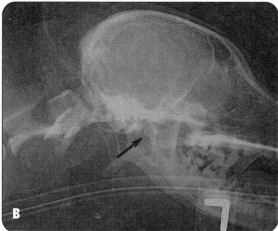

B

Figure 3-18

Lateral oblique technique for the temporomandibular joint in the dog (A). First the dog is placed in a straight lateral view. The beam is centered on the TMJ, just behind the angle of the mandible. Then the nose is lifted off of the table about 15 degrees, just enough to put the downside TMJ rostral to the cranium and isolating it on film (B, *see arrow*).

EXPOSING AND DEVELOPING THE FILM

As mentioned above, each dental film packet has a side that is to face toward the beam and one that is to face away. The side away from the beam is usually labeled with instructions molded into the plastic cover. If the molded letters were in the beam, they might show up on the image.

When taking several X rays, it is always prudent to place the exposed packets in one place and the unexposed in another. Some people like to use two jacket pockets; others put the exposed packets on the counter next to the developer or in some other special place. Unless there is blood or saliva on

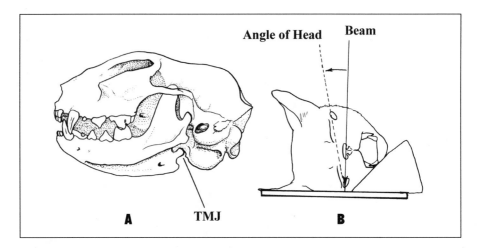

Figure 3-19

Lateral oblique technique for the temporomandibular joint in the cat.

(A) A view of the skull as if your eye were the beam. The beam is aimed between the two sides of the mandible, centered over where the TMJ is. In the cat, the temporo-mandibular joint slants down toward medial, rather than being straight across as in a dog.

(B) Positioning of the cat on the X-ray table. The cat is first placed with the head straight lateral. The head is then rolled top-foremost about 15 degrees toward the table with the beam aimed just above the angle of the mandible closest to the table.

the surface, exposed and unexposed packets are indistinguishable until, of course, they are developed. Everyone gets confused and occasionally develops unexposed or double-exposed film.

Intraoral films have a clever device for orienting you to which side of the mouth the X ray represents. On each packet a dimple is pressed into one corner from the back, which makes a visible and palpable mound on the film on

Figure 3-20

The film packet (and film inside) will have a dimple impressed into it. The resulting pimple should always be toward the X-ray source because there is a lead sheet on the opposite side. Since the pimple will distort the X-ray image somewhat, it should not cover the roots when the film is placed in the mouth. All intraoral X rays can easily be read if you remember that if the pimple faces you it is as if you are looking at the teeth from the outside of the mouth.

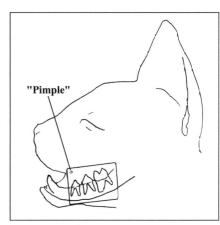

the side toward the beam (Fig. 3-20). When you look at the developed X ray, you will know that if the mound, or "pimple," faces you, you are looking at the correct side of the film. The dimple sometimes causes a distortion of the image, and occasionally a little light leaks into the packet because the plastic skin has been slightly torn when the dimple was made, thus exposing a small spot. The lesson here is that it is best to leave the dimple out of the image. One technique for this is to always put the dimple coronally, where it will cause little or no confusion. Another method is to always place the dimple in the same spot (i.e., lower right, for instance). However, in the final analysis, the dimple seldom causes serious problems in interpreting the X ray, and many people simply ignore where it is. In fact, it is one of the least important considerations for taking X rays.

Use of the Chairside Developer

The chairside developer (Fig. 3-21) has the capability of producing very accurate and artifact-free dental X rays, but it is somewhat technique sensitive (i.e., if the steps aren't followed correctly, the X ray suffers in quality), and its use

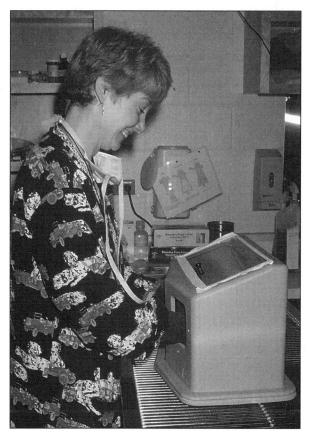

Figure 3-21

A chairside developer. The colored plastic top keeps out light that would expose the film yet allows the technician to see what he or she is doing.

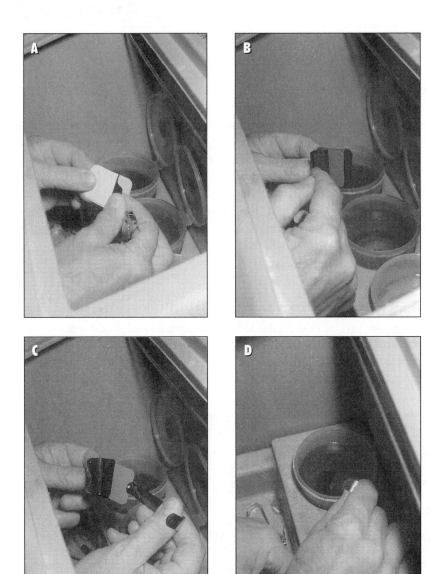

Figure 3-22

Developing film in the chairside developer.

(A) The film packet is opened inside the closed box. The clip should already be in the box so that the box can stay closed until the film is in the fixer.

(B) The film is isolated from covering paper and lead foil. It should be held only by the edges.

(C) The clip is attached securely to the film (if it is not secure, the film could come off in the solution container). To avoid placing it on the image, the clip should be attached to the end with the dimple/pimple.

(D) The film is put sequentially into developer, water rinse, fixer, and final water rinse, with the film left in each container, with adequate agitation, for the proper amount of time. The box may be opened after all open films are in the fixer or final rinse.

eats up personnel time. However, the steps are not difficult, and unless there is a high volume of dental X rays being taken, the expense of an automatic dental X-ray processor may not be justified. The time needed to develop dental X rays by hand approximates that of the automatic processor. Also, hand developing may yield quicker answers (to such questions as "did I get the apex?") because the "green" X ray forms an image in the developer in the first few seconds. Furthermore, automated processors may produce surface artifacts from contacts within the machine, or they may be excessively slow. The result is that for most practices hand developing in the chairside developer is standard.

The chairside developer is a box with holes for hands, a special orange-colored transparent plastic lid to watch what you are doing, and a series of four containers for developer, rinse, fixer, and second rinse. The hand holes are lined with a material that molds around the wrists or forearms to keep light out (it is usually spongy black neoprene, like wet suit material), and the orange blocks damaging light from the top. Like any X rays, dental X rays will react with light to completely expose the film and so must be developed in the "dark."

The developer and fixer for the chairside developer are special ultrafast chemicals made especially for this unit. They react within seconds with the film. The first step in developing films is to put whichever packets of film are to be processed inside the box along with a corresponding number of film clips. Then the top is closed, and via the hand holes, the plastic packet is opened inside the box (Fig. 3-22A). The film and lead foil are contained within a folded paper wrap under the plastic skin. The light green film is removed from the paper (only the edges of the film should be held) and attached to a clip (Figs. 3-22B and C). The film is immersed in the developer and agitated to get as much contact as possible with the chemical (Fig. 3-22D). If your fingers are contaminated with fixer, they can leave fingerprints or smudges on the film.

When the developer is fresh and relatively unused, the reaction of development will proceed rapidly, within a few seconds. As the developer gets "used up," the process will take longer. After swishing the film through the developer for about five seconds, it should be lifted out of the solution so that you can assess whether an image has appeared. It is dunked back in if it is still blank and reassessed every few seconds. As soon as an image appears in the film, it may be rinsed. It will not harm the film to allow it a couple more seconds in the developer, but if it is left too long, the film image will be lost to overdevelopment (the image will darken excessively).

The film is rinsed in plain water to remove the developer. It requires agitation for a solid 30 seconds. Next the film is put in the fixer. Up to this point the

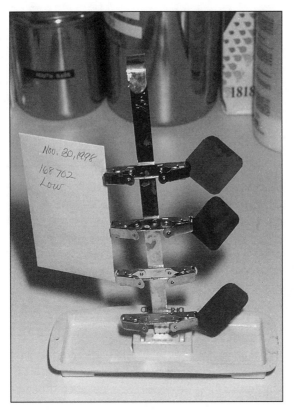

Figure 3-23

Small manilla envelope identifying case with corresponding films on drying stand. Each case should be identified from the start so that mixing of films does not occur. Once the films are dry, they can be placed in the envelope and filed.

film has a creamy, greenish, opaque surface, with the image appearing on top of it as if printed on light-colored paper. The fixer will eliminate the opaqueness and eventually cause the film to be clear except where the X rays have penetrated. The top of the developer can be opened as soon as the film enters the fixer, if desired. The film should stay in the fixer, with occasional agitation, until the film is entirely clear. Manufacturers usually recommend 30 to 45 seconds, but some people like to leave the film in it for a few minutes to be sure. Since this is a chemical reaction, and since chemical reactions are faster at higher temperatures, the process will depend on how warm or cold it is in the room. The chemical manufacturer's chart outlines recommended times for specific temperatures. Excessive time in the fixer can lead to bleaching of the film. The film can be taken wet from the fixer to be examined, if desired, and returned to finish fixing before rinsing.

The final rinse is plain water in which the film should be periodically agitated. The chemical manufacturer recommends a minimum of five minutes, but up to an hour will do no damage (longer may cause the emulsion to fall off the film). Good rinsing is the secret of "archival" quality in dental X rays. Any chemicals left on the film will cause degeneration of the film over weeks, months, or years. Both the first and second rinse baths should be refreshed after 5 to 15 X rays, depending on X-ray size. Typically, the first rinse takes on an orange or yellow hue when it has too much developer concentration in it, and although the fixer rinse will be clear, you can count on its concentration of chemical being too high to allow the film to rinse clean if the two containers have handled the same number of X rays.

If there are a lot of X rays to be done, the last rinse container can be made into a second fixer container, and the films set out on the counter to rinse in additional containers. Films can be damaged during processing by being scratched by other films or by getting stuck to other films in containers, so an increased number of containers in which the slower portions of the process occurs (fixing and postfixing rinsing) will make hand developing more efficient. Only the first three containers need be in the chairside developer box; the final rinse can be in normal light.

After the final rinse the film is hung up to dry. Films can be hung on their individual clips, or a multiple-clip unit can be utilized. These multiple-clip units can be used to separate cases during a busy X-ray day; the envelope for storage of the films, bearing the client's name and animal identification, can be suspended with the films or placed next to the holder (Fig. 3-23). Holders are made to hang or to be set on stands on a counter. The film should be placed in the holder clip by a corner, which will make another corner the lowest portion of the film. The water will then slide down and drip from that corner (it is easier for the water to drip from a corner than from an edge).

If the process of drying is too slow, you can touch an absorbent paper towel or tissue to the edge of the lower corner to wick excess water off the film. It is important not to try to wipe water off the surface of the film with anything, as wiping can damage the surface of the film and leave paper fibers on the slightly sticky, damp film surface. However, if paper fibers or fixer residues are obvious when the film is dry, they can be removed by rerinsing the film. Another method for rapidly removing water from the film is to blow it off with the air syringe from the dental unit or to use a hair dryer on a low- or no-heat setting.

Films should not be put into mounts or envelopes until completely dry because they will stick to the mounts or to each other and may be ruined. In humid climates, this may mean waiting hours until the surface is hard enough to store, unless artificial means of drying films (e.g., a hair dryer) are used. If there is adequate counter or hanging space, it may mean leaving films to dry overnight.

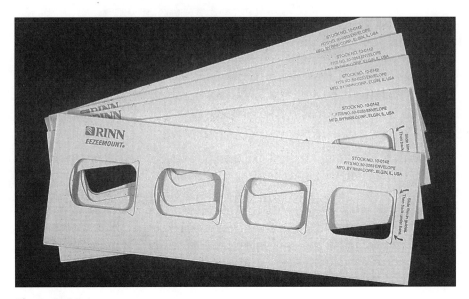

Figure 3-24

Film mounts are a convenient way to store films in their own folder or envelope.

STORAGE AND FILING OF DENTAL RADIOGRAPHS

Although there are tiny radiopaque numerals available for sticking onto dental X-ray packets, they are seldom used because they often get into the field of view. Because of their small size and lack of radiopaque markers, dates, or IDs, dental radiographs are easy to lose. There are several ways to file and retrieve films, which range from simple to elegant.

Radiographs should not be merely clipped or taped to the patient's file. Paper clips or staples will damage the film, and tape may leave residues that obstruct with the image or simply make it very difficult to take the film off the file to see what it shows. So the first thing that should be done is to develop an envelope system for the radiographs.

To store X rays, some people use the small manilla envelopes that are just larger than a number 4 film. A system can be developed whereby each X-ray visit rates an envelope, which is labeled with case number, last name, and date of visit. One animal might have several envelopes on file, which are arranged according to date. To avoid mixing the films when teeth are compared between visits, individual films can be labeled with the date and case number. A fine-tipped permanent marker should be used, and the film marked outside the image. The great disadvantage of this system is that the films are difficult

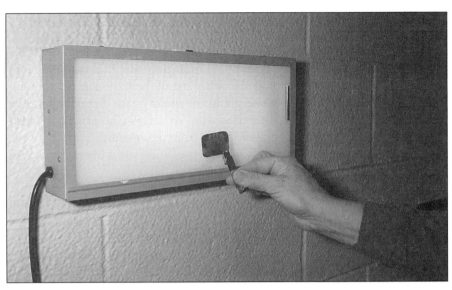

Figure 3-25
Dental X-ray viewer. Blocking out light around the film (as with a film mount) allows better visualization of the details on the film.

to view, and each time they are taken out, they must be oriented and what tooth or teeth are being looked at must be determined. Also, unless a black-out frame is used on the view box, the person looking at the film will be blinded by the light coming around the edges of the film. However, there is one major advantage to this system: it is space saving. This system is suited for a practice that does not take a lot of dental radiographs or one that has little space. Because films are separated by date of visit, the envelope method can easily be converted to a more involved system later on.

A more organized system utilizes film mounts (Fig. 3-24). Each visit merits a mount, or individual X rays taken on different dates can be grouped and labeled in a mount. Mounts are available in several configurations that correspond to film sizes for survey radiographs of cats or dogs, or they can be used to present individual radiographs in an organized way. The mount makes it easy to identify the animal and the time of the visit. Several mounts (realistically, the sum total of the animal's lifetime of dental radiographs) can be placed in a single 6 x 11-in. envelope. A mount is an attractive and professional way to organize and present radiographs. It makes viewing radiographs easier because it blocks bright light from the viewer (Fig. 3-25). There are several types of mounts available. They may be made of cardboard or plastic; some people prefer cardboard because it may be written on with a regular pen, whereas plastic requires a permanent marker.

OTHER SYSTEMS FOR DENTAL RADIOGRAPHY

Hand-held dental X-ray machines are now available, and although they cost roughly twice as much as a wall-mounted unit, they will find their way into practices. The main thing to remember with one of these units is not to point it at a person or to allow anyone to get in the direct beam. Being behind the unit, the operator will not usually expose him- or herself (this unit is designed to be held in both hands and pointed away from the operator), but there is a strong tendency, because the unit vaguely looks and points like a camera, to treat it with less respect than it deserves.

Self-developing dental X rays are presently being marketed. In combination with the hand-held X-ray unit, they could be very useful for a mobile practice—in zoo dentistry, for example. The packets are provided with an umbilicus into which chemicals are injected. X rays must be rinsed after development, but clips and flowing water or a rinse container are the only equipment needed. Of course, these packets are much more expensive than standard dental X rays, and the images may not be as sharp.

As discussed above, automatic film processors, similar to the processors found in many practices for larger X rays, are available for dental X rays. They have varying speeds of processing but do not provide the opportunity to glimpse the image seconds after the packet is opened. Most seem to take 90 seconds to five minutes from start to finish, and the packet must still be opened by hand in a box. Noncontact processors are probably slower but will avoid artifacts caused by the film touching a carrier surface. They are not inexpensive but are useful when large numbers of survey radiographs are made.

Probably the newest technology available is digital dental radiology. More likely to be found in a university or research setting, these units cost as much as a small automobile. A sensitive plate attached to the computer replaces dental films, and the computer stores each image it is asked to keep. The digitally stored X rays can be kept on the computer or a disc, or they can be printed out, and the hard copies stored. You can imagine a disc containing all the radiographs taken over a patient's lifetime—it is an elegant storage solution.

INTERPRETATION OF DENTAL RADIOGRAPHS

Dental radiographs are essentially the same as any other X rays in that different densities of tissues block X rays to a greater or lesser extent. When the rays pass through no tissue, they completely expose the film and show up as pure black. Soft tissues, either fat, skin, or muscle, show up as a "water" density, or a very dark gray; generally the thicker these tissues are, the lighter the gray because fewer rays are able to penetrate the tissue. Bone density is a light gray, because the calcified tissues allow few rays through; and teeth, which are a modified dense bone, appear even whiter. Pure white forms are found when metal, like lead or steel, blocks all X rays from striking the film. Barium is an element that blocks X rays very effectively, and it is used for contrast studies in the GI tract and to make dental materials show up better on radiographs (like gutta-percha, which is used to fill root canals). When a substance blocks X rays, it is called radiodense, or radiopaque, and the more radiopaque it is, the easier it is to see. As with soft tissue, bone and teeth may overlap, and the more layers there are, the more radiopaque they show. Superimposing structures may interfere with interpretation, just as you may not recognize a friend if someone is standing in front of him!

TROUBLESHOOTING

As a technician, you will not be expected to interpret pathology on X rays—that is the responsibility of the veterinarian. However, you will need to be able to produce radiographs that are diagnostic. The veterinarian can see the crown with his or her own eyes; what the veterinarian cannot see are the roots. So the object of dental radiographs is to produce as true an image of the roots as possible. One way to provide the least distortion is to place the film as close to the subject as is practical. However, large films may be prevented from (for instance) being placed against the palate because of tooth crowns. If tooth crowns are pushing the edges of the packet away from the palate, resist the temptation to bend the film. This will almost certainly result in distortion of the image. Using the smallest film possible is one way to get around the distortion caused by bent film.

Since the root is the important part of the X ray, you may wish to sacrifice the image of the crown for the root. This is especially true of the canines, whose banana shape can cause confusion about the long axis of the tooth. If the axis of the root is used as the target, the crown portion may be quite foreshortened —but who cares?

If the portion of the final X ray that strikes the film with no tissue interposed is not black, the film has not been exposed adequately or has not been in the developer long enough. This may be an indication that the chemicals should be changed. Similarly, if the fixer does not clear the film within about 30 seconds, the fixer is exhausted. Although the chemicals can sometimes be used for many more films than the manufacturer recommends, if the times for developing and fixing lengthen, the chemicals should be replaced regardless of whether the chemicals have "just been changed." Chemicals should never be diluted with water, even if evaporation is suspected—they should be changed. In regions in which tap water is contaminated with minerals (hard water), it may be preferable to rinse with distilled water.

Smudges or scratches on the X rays represent handling problems during development. In extremely dry periods when static electricity readily occurs, it is possible (although rare) to have a static discharge occur across a film packet. This will appear as a "lightning" tracing across the film. Amalgam or barium in the animal's tissues or hair will produce white marks. If the film packet is inadvertently exposed through the foil (through the wrong side), the film will be less distinct and will sometimes show a stippled or grid pattern from the foil. If film has been partially exposed (for instance, if it is left on the counter and stray radiation contacts it), it may be darker than normal—or if only part of the film packet was exposed, it may have a darker portion that corresponds to the edge of whatever was on top of it (usually another film). If stray light gets into the chairside developer, the edge of the foil layer or plastic cover may show up on a film where it blocked the light.

If a technician can produce films without artifacts, with good visualization of the roots, and with minimal distortion, the veterinarian will have a powerful diagnostic tool for complete dental care.

Periodontal Disease

Periodontal disease is far and away the most frequent cause of loss of teeth in cats and dogs. Certainly there are teeth lost to resorptive lesions in cats (which could be considered a subcategory of periodontal disease—see below). Fractures in both species can eventually result in the loss of teeth because of the development of endodontal disease. A few dogs have caries ("cavities") that can destroy teeth. Yet most teeth are lost because of the destruction of the supporting structures of the teeth, not because of pathology in the teeth themselves.

THE DEVELOPMENT OF PERIODONTAL DISEASE

The Role of Plaque

Periodontal means "around the teeth," and periodontal disease is disease of the gingiva (gums), periodontal ligament, and bone. As we all know from television and print advertisements, periodontal disease begins with that evil entity, plaque. The progression of periodontal disease is the same for animals as people, so what is said about humans goes for animals as well (Fig. 4-1). Without plaque, animals and people would never have periodontitis, mainly because they would be dead.

Plaque consists of three main elements. The first is bacteria. We (animals and ourselves) could probably live without bacteria in our mouths—in fact, we did before birth—but it would not be long before more bacteria would be introduced from food, the pencil we hold in our mouth, the attractive person we kiss on a date, or licking our feet or backside (in the case of cats and dogs). Some of the bacteria we take into our mouths is benign; it will not hurt us because it is basically noninvasive, the stomach will take care of most bacteria with its acid bath, or we already have a degree of immunity to it. The normal bacteria of the mouth is considered nonpathological, like the normal bacteria on our skin.

People have essentially the same bacteria in their mouths as cats and dogs do. There are different species of bacteria for different species of animals, but they are of the same general type. The normal oral flora consists of aerobic (i.e., thriving in the presence of oxygen) small coccoid (round) gram-positive (meaning the mucopolysaccharide bacterial wall stains with Gram's stain) bacteria. Normal oral bacteria are beneficial because their presence inhibits other microorganisms, like disease-causing bacteria or fungi, from becoming established.

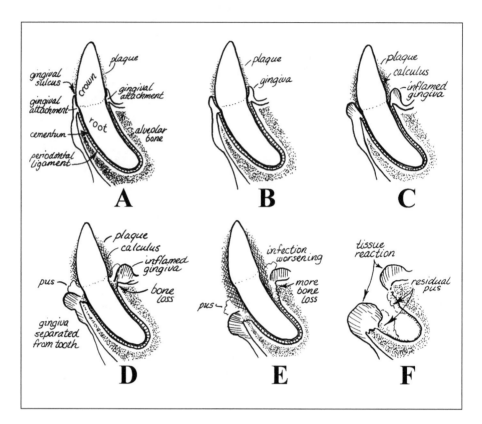

Figure 4-1

Progression of periodontal disease.

(A and B) Plaque is the inciting entity in periodontal disease. If plaque is not regularly cleaned off teeth, the bacteria it contains multiply.

(C) In addition, after about two days plaque begins to mineralize into calculus. Dental calculus is porous and contains a thriving population of bacteria; it is also mechanically irritating to soft tissues. Inflammation of the gingiva (gingivitis) with reddening and swelling is the first sign of periodontitis.

(D and E) Colonization of the gingival sulcus with anaerobic bacteria starts the process of attachment loss because the bacteria and their by-products cause the deterioration of soft tissues and then bone.

(F) When attachment loss of the periodontal ligament reaches a certain stage, the tooth becomes loose and eventually exfoliates (falls out).

The second component of plaque is saliva. Saliva provides the moist environment that allows the bacteria to live.

The third component is food, which nourishes bacteria as well as ourselves. That is why we would have to be dead if we didn't have plaque—because, like bacteria, we could not live without eating.

The Dynamics of Bacterial Proliferation

Although the normal flora is considered benign, if the numbers of bacteria are allowed to get too large, they can cause damage to periodontal tissues. Because of the slimy, mucoid nature of saliva, and because of the slimy mucopolysaccharides produced by live, vegetative (actively growing) bacteria, plaque sticks to teeth. If plaque isn't removed from teeth and swallowed (this is happening to a certain degree constantly as saliva bathes our mouths) and the source of nourishment is steady, the numbers of bacteria increase exponentially. Bacteria multiply by dividing in two. If you had one bacterium with plenty of nourishment, in a few minutes you would have two in the next generation, four in the next, eight in the next, then sixteen, thirty-two, and so on. Needless to say, you would soon have a lot of bacteria. In fact, in about two days the average person or animal would have enough bacteria to cause inflammation of the gingiva.

As bacterial numbers in the plaque increase, the thickness of the plaque increases on the tooth. At the same time, the high numbers of bacteria are producing metabolites (waste materials), mainly acids, which can have a direct effect on the gingiva and teeth. More sugar in the diet results in more acid, which can eat the surface enamel off the teeth and then start on the dentin underneath (which is caries). The reason humans as a group get caries and dogs and cats as a group do not is that these animals have a great deal less refined sugar in their diets. (The reason adult humans have less caries than children is that normal adults develop a partial immunity to the bacteria as they age.)

The word *caries*, by the way, is a Latin noun meaning "decay" or "rottenness." It is not plural in meaning, and to say "a carie" is absolutely incorrect. If it is uncomfortable to say "a caries," you can speak or write about "a carious lesion."

Undisturbed plaque undergoes two changes with time. One change is that minerals in the saliva, especially calcium, impregnate the soft plaque matrix and cause it to gradually harden into dental calculus, the common name of which is tartar. In addition, the dominant type of bacteria tends to change as periodontal disease progresses. The thicker plaque and calcifying plaque tend to shield bacteria from air and oxygen, and a different population of bacteria begins to proliferate—anaerobic rods and spirochetes, which are generally gram-negative and disease causing. As soon as this population takes over, periodontitis begins in earnest.

Gingivitis, the First Sign of Periodontitis

The acids and other by-products of metabolism of the normal flora, when produced in abundance, can cause a reaction in the gingiva. The first area to be affected is that part directly adjacent to the plaque—the leading edge of the

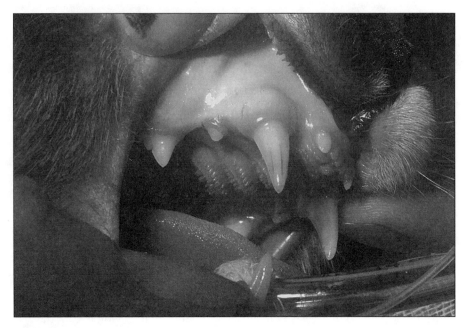

Figure 4-2

Marginal (at the free gingival margin) gingivitis in a cat. The dark margin indicates that, although teeth do not appear to have calculus in place, inflammation is already well advanced.

free gingival margin (Fig. 4-2). Its reaction is to redden and swell, which is caused by the tissue mobilizing an increased blood supply with white cells (chiefly the phagocytic neutrophil) to fight the invading bacteria. This process is triggered by the presence of the chemicals released by the bacteria and those released by the tissues as they respond to the bacteria. The new population of pathogenic bacteria accelerates this process.

As marginal gingivitis occurs and the edge of the free gingival margin begins to swell, it loses its ability to cling to the tooth surface like thin rubber on a bathtub. In addition, the sulcular epithelium will exude antibody and neutrophil-rich fluid to stop the attack of the bacteria; this defense tends to lift the sulcular epithelium off the tooth surface. As a result of relentless attack on the gingiva without periodic removal of plaque and calculus, bacterial colonies, then plaque and calculus, are established underneath the marginal gingiva. The anaerobic bacteria are now free to attack the attachments of the tooth. Gingivitis like this is stage 1 of periodontitis (PDI 1) and is totally reversible.

Attachment Loss Begins

The first tissues to be attacked and destroyed are the fibers of the attached gingiva at the CEJ (cemento-enamel junction). Once bacteria infect these tissues, the attachments are assaulted by the bacteria's destructive capabilities combined with the autolytic (tissue-dissolving) enzymes of the neutrophils responding to their presence. The tissues become necrotic (die) and serve as nourishment for the bacteria that thrive in dead tissue (usually rods and spirochetes). True tooth attachment has now been lost; this is full-blown periodontal disease. Soft tissue is more susceptible to necrosis than bone, so the next area to suffer is the periodontal ligament and the cementum covering the root. As the ligament is destroyed, adjacent bone is also affected to a lesser extent. The infection proceeds apically (toward the root tip), and periodontal pockets are formed.

Periodontal pockets are palpatable attachment losses beyond the CEJ that extend under gingiva more than 4 mm in dogs and 2 mm in cats or that extend beyond the attached gingiva into the mucosa. Part of the technician's job in performing a dental prophy (cleaning) is to find and document the position and depth of periodontal pockets and to clean them out with closed root planing if possible (see Chap. 5).

Further Progression of Periodontal Disease

The gingiva responds in two possible ways to periodontal disease: recession (loss) or hyperplasia (abnormal and excessive growth). In most animals the response is to recede (Fig. 4-3). The gingiva, although still inflamed, loses tissue at the free gingival margin, and the total width of the attached gingiva is reduced. This mainly occurs when there is extensive bone loss under the gingiva and there is no longer bone to support it. Finally, in an advanced case, the gingiva is completely destroyed, and the lesion continues all the way to the mucosa. This carries a very grim prognosis for the tooth because mucosa will not form a barrier to plaque and bacteria since it does not make a tight attachment to the bone. Only with grafting of new attached gingiva (if possible) will this tooth have a chance for long-term retention; otherwise, the progressive infection will resume unabated under the mucosa.

When the loss of attachment of the periodontal ligament progresses far enough apically, the tooth becomes loose. Typically, two-thirds of the periodontal ligament must be destroyed before a tooth shows movement, but this differs by the tooth. Obviously, a small, single-rooted tooth, like the first premolar in a dog, is more likely to move than an upper fourth premolar, particularly if only one of the three roots of the larger tooth has periodontal loss of attachment. As a rule, *any* movement of a tooth with more than one root spells extraction because it takes extensive periodontal ligament and bone destruction to effect displacement.

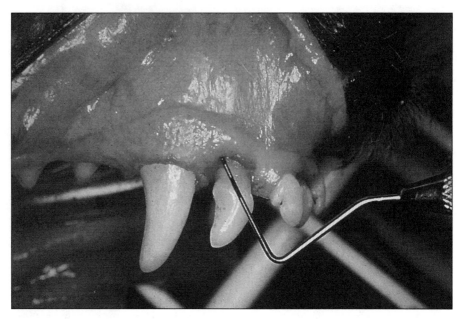

Figure 4-3

Recession of bone and gingiva, exposing the tooth roots, is the most frequent manifestation of periodontitis in cats and is often seen in dogs as well. The root is narrower than the crown, but the teeth have an enamel bulge under the gum line adjacent to the root, so any time the tooth narrows next to the gum line, there has been gingival recession.

There is an exception to the general indication that movement is due to periodontitis. The lower incisors may show slight or even advanced movement without signs of periodontal pockets or even inflammation of the gingiva. What is going on here? This phenomenon, sometimes called periodontosis, is usually seen in small dogs; it occurs because there is so little space between the roots of the incisors that the bone doesn't form effective alveoli for the teeth. In radiographs, these teeth appear to be floating in space. The teeth are useless and will exfoliate (come out) easily because they are merely anchored by the gingiva. They can be retained for aesthetic reasons with an orthodontic technique called periodontal splinting (see Chap. 11).

The Impact of Periodontal Infection

Periodontitis that results in loose teeth is a serious infection. One result of the infection and destruction is very obvious: oral malodor, or halitosis. There are people who think their dog or cat has bad breath who are smelling only cat or dog food or something else the animal has ingested (which, especially in dogs who eat carrion or cat excrement, can be really foul). The characteristic odor of severe periodontitis is that of rotting meat because similar bacteria are "rotting" the periodontal tissues. Not surprisingly, these animals are in distress. The inflammation of the gingiva and mucosa alone will be painful, not to mention the deep infection in the bone. Another characteristic of deep periodontal infections is the very dark color of the necrotic tissues, which can even appear black due to bacterial pigmentation.

Every time a dog or cat with moderate or severe periodontitis eats, the animal is causing abrasions to fragile infected gingiva, bone, or oral mucosa. When the tissues tear, as they will undoubtedly do, capillaries will rupture, and there will be bleeding. The presence of bacteria in the blood is called septicemia, and transient septicemias occur all the time in periodontitis patients. What happens to the bacteria liberated into the bloodstream? It largely depends on numbers and on the ability of the host to defend itself (the immune system). An animal with a weakened immune system will be much more susceptible to invasion by septicemic bacteria. Things that can weaken immunity include stress, immunosuppressive drugs like those given for cancer or certain autoimmune diseases, metabolic diseases and other infections, neoplasms (cancers), poor body condition, and so on. (These factors are discussed in more detail in Chap. 6.)

A small amount of bacteria in the blood is rapidly cleaned up by white blood cells. Actually, the body is set up for small numbers of bacteria to challenge its defenses. Bacteria in the gut are fairly routinely liberated into the bloodstream in tiny numbers and are rapidly cleaned up as they are filtered by the liver. Bacteria released by periodontitis, however, may go to any part of the body after leaving the mouth; first to the heart, from the cranial vena cava; then to the lungs; then to high–blood-flow organs like the kidneys. In fact, infections of the kidneys have been statistically related to periodontitis in dogs, and no doubt as methods of investigation become more sophisticated, infections of other organs will be documented as well.

In humans endocarditis (infection of the inner lining of the heart, especially the valves) has been found to be caused by periodontitis-induced septicemia. Therefore, people with heart conditions that might make them susceptible to endocarditis are given antibiotics when they get their teeth cleaned to avoid showers of bacteria as their gingivae are traumatized.

Recently even mild human periodontitis was linked to conditions as unlikely as low–birth-weight babies. There have been many anecdotal accounts of periodontitis leading to other serious disease in animals, and it only makes sense. A person or an animal would have to incur a horrible filthy wound to allow enough bacteria to invade the body to become septicemic, and then, most likely either the body would find a way to wall off the infection or the

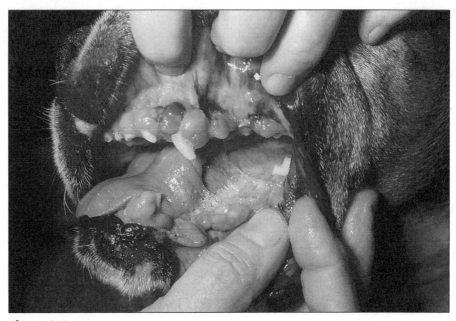

Figure 4-4
Another response to gingival inflammation seen more often in dogs than in cats is gingival hyperplasia. The irritated gingiva proliferates, sometimes until the teeth are buried in thick, tumorous-looking gingiva. The dog pictured is a boxer, one of the breeds very prone to this condition.

body would die. Unfortunately, there is no way to wall off the mouth, and periodontitis progresses until the teeth are exfoliated and the periodontal tissues can heal. Yet in the process, the host suffers.

GINGIVAL HYPERPLASIA

There are some interesting twists to periodontitis. One is the way in which the gingiva sometimes reacts even to mild inflammation. Usually seen in dogs, rarely in cats, gingival hyperplasia, or hypertrophy, is a sort of runaway growth of gingiva (Fig. 4-4). The free gingival margin lengthens and distorts, sometimes making tumorous-looking growths, and in the process creating what are called pseudopockets. These pockets get their depth from the lengthening of the margin, not from loss of attachment beyond the CEJ (although there can be, and often is, attachment loss in addition to the gingival hyperplasia). If the hyperplasia is perpetuated, the length of the pocket will allow pathogenic bacteria to establish themselves in the sulcus, and very quickly the process of attachment loss will occur. The treatment for gingival hyperplasia is amputation, called a gingivoplasty (see Chap. 9).

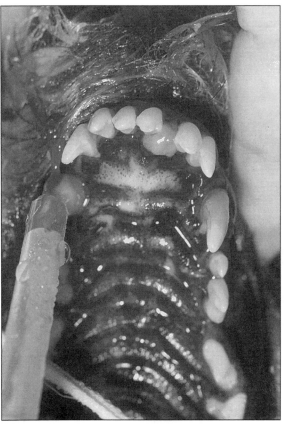

Figure 4-5
Single oral masses without other instances of gingival hyperplasia are suspicious of cancer, especially if the surface looks different from surrounding gingiva or mucosa or if teeth are displaced by the mass.

Oral Masses

A note about gingival hyperplasia is in order here. Hyperplasia is always connected to the attached gingiva, and its surface is identical to attached gingiva. If the surface of a mass is of a different color or texture from the gingiva, a tumor should be suspected (Fig. 4-5). If bone is affected (either increased, as a lump, or decreased, which is usually only evident as a lysis or decrease in bone density in a radiograph), a tumor is very likely. Neoplasms (cancers) can look like severe inflammation, and if inflammation seems excessive for the amount of calculus and attachment loss, a tumor is a likely cause. Excessive inflammation may also be due to autoimmune causes. Deciding how much inflammation to expect with a certain degree of calculus is a matter of experience. Fortunately, that experience will come rapidly as you look at many mouths.

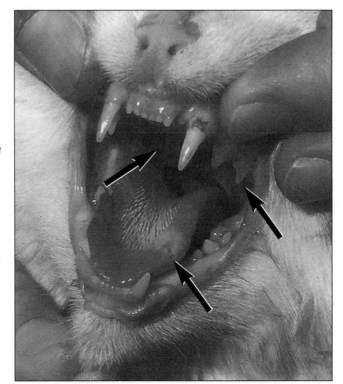

Figure 4-6

Some cats are subject to a painful condition called feline stomatitis. In response to the bacteria present around the teeth, the cat's body seems to have an allergic reaction to the tissues lining the mouth, which become very painful and friable. This particular cat had lesions on its tongue as well as the mucosa in the rear of the mouth (see arrows).

FELINE STOMATITIS

A painful and sometimes devastating condition sometimes seen in cats, stomatitis is an inflammation of the mouth that can become so severe that the cat will refuse to take anything orally (Fig. 4-6). It tends to be mainly in the caudal mouth, where it can be called faucitis (for inflammation of the fauces, the pharyngeal arch just behind the teeth), or it can appear to be limited to the gingiva. However, many unfortunate cats, particularly purebreds, have a generalized stomatitis.

The feline stomatitis syndrome is caused by the bacteria that inhabit the cat's mouth and by the cat's immune response to them. The only place bacteria have access to the soft tissue blood supply is in the sulci of the attached gingiva; the rest of the gingiva and oral mucosa, if intact, makes an effective barrier to the blood. It is not known why some cats have such a severe reaction to their oral bacteria or the bacteria's metabolites. However, in affected cats, a huge influx of the white blood cells most active in immune processes (lymphocytes and plasmacytes) occurs, and the soft tissues become very reddened and friable. In fact, color and consistency resemble that of strawberry jelly.

A cat that has routine periodontitis due to dirty teeth may become quite uncomfortable and resemble a stomatitis cat. The diseases are differentiated by two things: (1) The condition of the cat without stomatitis will resolve after cleaning (and extractions, if needed) whereas that of the stomatitis cat will not, and (2) a biopsy of the tissue will show the presence or absence of lymphocytes and plasmacytes. A reasonable course of treatment would be a thorough prophy first with a biopsy at the same time or at a later date if the mouth doesn't improve.

Because lymphocytic/plasmacytic gingivitis (or stomatitis, if it is more generalized in the mouth) is caused by an excessive immune response to the oral flora, the treatment is to reduce the numbers of bacteria, suppress the immune response, or both. Antibiotics active against a broad spectrum of bacteria or oral disinfectant rinses can reduce the bacterial burden. The obvious immunosuppressant drugs (corticosteroids) can be used, or there are more exotic immune modulators like gold salts that have been successful. Another route is to rid the mouth of the source of access to the bloodstream, the gingival sulci, by extracting the teeth. If the condition is mainly around the caudal teeth, the rostral teeth may be spared. However, full-mouth extraction is considered a cure for the condition. Although it has been reported that extractions have not cured stomatitis, this is questionable: there was probably something else going on, such as retained, infected tooth roots or sharp alveolar edges causing continuing inflammation. Cats do not need teeth to eat commercial cat foods, so they get along beautifully without a single tooth and are comfortable at last.

Occasionally a diffuse squamous cell carcinoma can mimic stomatitis. The cancer obviously would have a grave prognosis.

Dogs may rarely have a similar condition or be suffering from oral pemphigus vulgaris or other autoimmune diseases. The key is to biopsy lesions so that an informed treatment plan can be devised.

FELINE RESORPTIVE LESIONS

Some cats, for reasons unknown, have a devastating response to inflammation due to even mild periodontitis: feline resorptive lesions (or FORL, for feline odontoclastic resorptive lesion). These lesions, once called "cat cavities," are not caries at all but the result of attack by remodeling bone cells called osteoclasts (Fig. 4-7). Bone is constantly remodeling itself; the single osteoclasts eat their way through old bone and are followed by the osteoblasts, which form new bone in the tunnel excavated for them. The new bone is called the osteoid seam. Feline osteoclasts, apparently turned on by inflammation, migrate from the edge of the alveolar bone to attack the tooth (which, after

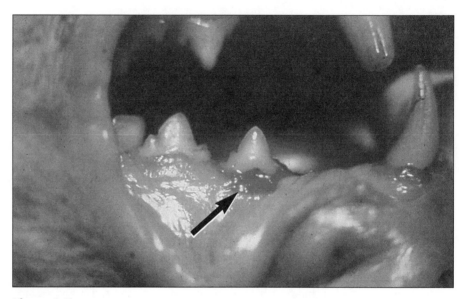

Figure 4-7
Feline resorptive lesions occur when bone-dissolving osteoclast cells from the alveolar bone respond to periodontal inflammation by attacking the dentin at the cemento-enamel junction. The cat's gingiva often tries to cover up the hole in the tooth with a dark bleb of tissue.

all, is modified bone) at the CEJ. The destruction of the tooth is usually quite rapid; from the first indication of resorption to perforation of the pulp can be as little as a few months.

There are several characteristics of resorptive lesions. One is that, unlike caries, the concavities at the neck of the teeth are cleanly excavated; they lack the soft deteriorated dentinal margins and dark decayed debris of caries. Another characteristic, shared with caries, is that these teeth are sensitive. Rapid erosion into the dentin has decreased the dentinal insulation to the sensitive pulp, and pain is the result. Cats often salivate profusely, resist having their cheeks touched, and may even stop eating. And finally, these lesions often have a characteristic glistening red bleb of inflamed gingiva over them, which probably acts as a sort of bandage over the sensitive pulp. Rather than being on the lingual (tongue) or palatal side, they are usually on the buccal (cheek) or labial (lip) side of the teeth because this is where periodontal inflammation is more likely to begin, where the raspy tongue is not constantly wiping the teeth. At the CEJ, osteoblasts do not follow the osteoclasts, probably because the environment (air and saliva) are not conducive to their functioning. Deep in the bone, however, resorptive lesions can result in the remodeling of dentin to bone.

Resorptive lesions are classed 1, 2, or 3 according to their depth. If, when palpated, they are found to be only as deep as the enamel, which is less than a millimeter in cats, they are reported as a 1. Those that have attacked the dentin but have not perforated the pulp are a 2. Those that invade the pulp are a 3. Shallow resorptive lesions are difficult to assess visually. A dental explorer is needed to palpate the slight edge of enamel that always accompanies a resorptive lesion of the crown. If simple gingival recession exposed the divots of the furcations between the roots, these should be palpated. Furcations without resorptive lesions feel like smooth depressions. Radiographs will show loss of tooth structure whether it is in the crown or, as occasionally happens, mainly or entirely in the root.

The prognosis for resorptive lesions is grim. Although some practitioners still attempt to place restorations in resorptive lesions, studies and observations have shown that most of these are doomed to fail in just a few months. Perforation of the pulp spells death to the tooth, and the small size of the teeth usually affected does not allow endodontal therapy. If teeth with painful resorptive lesions are not extracted, the lesions inevitably progress, and eroded crowns snap off with sharp shards left at the gum line. In most cases the gingiva covers over these shards, but whenever the cat bites down on anything firm, pain results. There may be tiny ulcers over the retained roots from endodontal infection or simply from trauma.

If the retained roots are not painful or causing ulcerated gingiva, they may safely be allowed to remain but should be removed if they are causing pathology. Retained roots can be identified by bumps in the alveolar crest and by X ray. Occasionally, if they continue to be resorbed, they will leave a strangely mottled bone behind in their absence, which will show up on an X ray.

Dogs may show a similar pathology, called external resorptive lesions, in tooth roots. These are usually an endodontal condition.

THE HEALING POWER OF THE PERIODONTIUM

In early periodontitis, when gingivitis is present but attachment loss of gingiva or bone has not occurred, the inflammation can be completely reversed by cleaning the crowns of the teeth, which allows the gingiva to resume normal shape and function once the calculus and bacteria are removed. Once attachment loss or gingival recession has occurred, however, the chances of complete return to normal periodontium diminishes.

A shallow periodontal pocket, without the loss of bone, will resolve with complete cleaning of the tooth, bone, gingival sulcular space, and pocket surfaces.

However, once bone is destroyed, it never comes back by itself. If the surface of the root has been cleaned, it can act like cortical bone, and the gingiva may form attachments to it, but the dentin is denser than bone and probably does not allow as tight an attachment as bone does. Plus the bone itself must taper gradually to a point, with no necrotic bone present, so in order to reform an attachment, the bone itself must be remodeled by the dental surgeon if it ends abruptly (the technique of removing bone to make a better contour is called osteoplasty).

Pocket depth can be reduced by use of a localized antibiotic treatment deep in the tissues (Heska perioceutic). New bone may be induced to grow in a pocket by a process called guided tissue regeneration. In this technique, pockets are surgically opened, a matrix material, either transplanted cancellous bone or an artificial product, is placed where the bone is desired, and the gingiva is closed over it. This is a rare technique in veterinary medicine because it requires a great deal of aftercare, and veterinary patients can be noncooperative. Another "salvage" technique is the creation of apically repositioned flaps. Here the attached gingiva and mucosa are undermined and moved across bone so they can reattach farther beyond the tooth crown on bone. Assisting in these techniques is discussed in Chapter 9.

All periodontal care is time-intensive in the original therapy and in the maintenance afterward. Unfortunately, the result is always less functional than the original. Exposed dentin in roots is sensitive until odontoblasts fill in dentinal tubules because root dentin is normally covered by bone. When bone and gingiva recede, the enamel bulge is destroyed and no longer deflects food off the teeth during chewing. Instead of a bulge where gingiva meets the crown, an indentation occurs between the crown and the root. Food and plaque accumulate in this depression, exacerbating the progression of periodontal disease.

The best therapy for periodontal disease is prevention. Here is where the dental technician may provide the most service to clients and their animals through the dental prophy and client education.

Performing the Dental Prophy

The dental prophy (which is short for *prophylaxis*, meaning "preventative") is so named because removal of dental calculus will *prevent* progression of periodontal disease. The dental prophy is usually performed by the veterinary technician. Its purpose is to clean the teeth thoroughly. It could be called a dental cleaning, not a "dental" (even though this is how it's commonly referred to in veterinary clinics). This is because the word *dental* is only an adjective, like hairy, and it needs a noun to modify. *Dental prophy* is preferred.

SAFETY AND HEALTH CONSIDERATIONS

Before beginning a prophy, you should give some thought to animal and personnel safety. A first concern is that the animal's gingiva will be traumatized during the prophy, usually causing bleeding. Bleeding signals an opening into the circulatory system, and if blood can escape, bacteria can (and do) enter the circulation. The animal can usually take care of a small amount of bacteria. After all, whenever it gets a scratch, bacteria enter the bloodstream. In a younger animal with very little bacterial growth in its mouth, the trauma from a prophy would probably amount to very little potential for problems, as is the case with most people who get their teeth cleaned. However, many animals who come in for a prophy are there because they have a foul-smelling, dirty mouth, which means huge amounts of infection. Even if the mouth doesn't look too bad, all animals should be protected by an antibiotic in the bloodstream at the time of the procedure (Fig. 5-1).

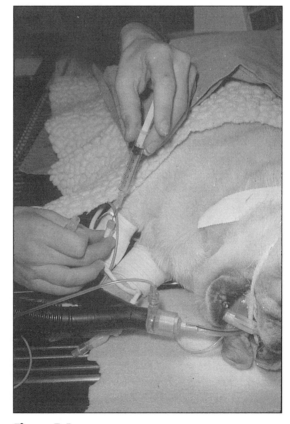

Figure 5-1

Administering antibiotics intravenously. The presence of antibiotics is critical to the comfort and well-being of the patient undergoing even a routine dental prophy.

The antibiotic can then kill bacteria before they have a chance to set up a hematogenous (blood-borne) infection in an organ. It is much more difficult to treat an infection than to prevent one.

If oral antibiotics are used, they should be administered several hours prior to the procedure. The optimal time is probably equivalent to one-half of the dose interval before beginning. For instance, if the drug is normally given every six hours, it should be given three hours before the prophy. This is because in the middle of the dosing cycle the antibiotic should be at full blood level. Oral antibiotics have their drawbacks, however, not the least of which is the talent some animals have of spitting them out. The absorption rate of the drug and the time it takes to get into the bloodstream can be affected by several factors as well.

Injectable antibiotics are preferable for these reasons. Subcutaneous or intramuscular antibiotics are probably in the bloodstream within an hour, but if the animal is cold and circulation is stagnant, their spread will be delayed. This is why I prefer intravenous drugs. As soon as they are given, the animal will have a protective level of antibiotic in circulation. Unfortunately, some antibiotics (e.g., penicillin) cannot be administered intravenously (IV).

The type of antibiotic is not as important as making sure that (1) it is as broad a spectrum (kills as wide a variety of bacteria) as possible, (2) it will be in the blood when it is needed, and (3) it is given appropriately. Even rather narrow-spectrum drugs, such as penicillin, are effective even though they might not be able to fight an established infection of the same bacteria.

Other patient support procedures are included in Chapter 6.

The location in the clinic for the dental prophy should be a designated "dirty" area. Ultrasonic or other power scalers cause billions of bacteria to be aerosolized as teeth are cleaned, and these settle on counters, walls, and other surfaces. Obviously, this should not be allowed in a surgical suite or near an intensive care block of cages. Dental prophies can be performed in common areas that are used for tasks such as toenail clipping, bathing, and other routine procedures; prophies do not have to have an area devoted strictly to them (although a dedicated area is preferable for the sake of convenience and the above reasons).

Besides the health and safety of patients, there are also important considerations for the staff. First, aerosolized bacteria can potentially affect humans. The bacteria from a dirty mouth can cause skin, eye, nose and throat, or lung infections if inhaled. So one form of safety equipment you should wear is a surgical mask. Aerosolization of bacteria from power scaling generally occurs within 3 ft of the animal's head, and anyone within this zone should wear a mask (Fig. 5-2).

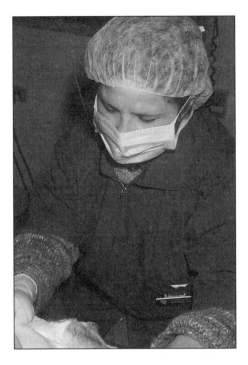

Figure 5-2

The technician should protect him- or herself with a mask and face shield or glasses from the aerosolized or spattering bacteria. Shown here is a combination mask/face shield that is disposable.

The next safety item that should always be in place is eye protection. Sprays from the mouth, calculus snapped off teeth, broken or loose burs from high-speed drills all have the potential for entering your eye and injuring or infecting it. The minimum eye protection is a pair of eyeglasses (with impact-resistant plastic lenses) or simple goggles. However, neither of these protect your face from flying debris, so a clear face mask is preferable. There are some face masks that fasten around the head at the forehead that can easily be worn with a surgical mask underneath them; they have another advantage in that they do not fog up like eyeglasses or goggles do when worn with a surgical mask. There are also styles of disposable face shields that are connected to a surgical mask.

There are certain mouths that are cesspools of infection that you would be loathe to put your bare hands into for multiple hygienic reasons. Bacterial contamination can set up an infection in a scratch or hangnail. Also, not only could you introduce infective agents into your mouth (even after washing) when eating but the odor of decay that may cling to your hands could cause loss of appetite. Therefore, cultivate the habit of wearing exam gloves, if only for the more disgusting cases.

Last, you could make an argument for wearing surgical caps and other dedicated clothing during dental prophies. You are in a cloud of bacteria during the prophy. It would be prudent not to carry this bacteria home or to the next patient.

SETTING UP FOR A SIMPLE PROPHYLAXIS

A minimum of equipment is needed for the basic prophy. A power scaler (preferably ultrasonic) and polisher speed up the procedure and make it more professional. (See Chap. 2 for comparisons of different types of equipment.) You should also have a few hand instruments. These should include something to crack thick calculus off teeth, such as a calculus forceps or an extraction forceps. You should have a periodontal probe, with or without a dental explorer. For getting intractable chips of calculus off tooth crowns, especially in the divots and grooves that the ultrasonic scaler can't reach, you will want a scaler. Finally, you will want a curette to pass under the gum line to assure yourself that you have removed any and all calculus there. A mouth gag is not absolutely necessary but makes access to the teeth easier. Disposable mouth props can be made from recycled syringe barrels or covers as well as catheter covers.

There are a few necessary supplies also. A water source (preferably an air/water syringe) washes away blood and debris so that you can see the teeth. Gauze sponges are convenient for wiping teeth or gums and for placing in the pharynx (the back of the mouth) to keep debris away from the larynx. (Note that it is *critical* to remove the gauze sponge before the animal is recovered because it could suffocate the animal if it is left in place.) A polishing compound, or "prophy paste," may be bought in bulk or in individual portions. Buying individual portions will prevent contamination between animals. An oral disinfectant as a rinse kills bacteria when it is applied before or after cleaning.

PERFORMING THE PROPHY, STEP BY STEP

Once the animal is on the table and anesthetized, a few tasks should be performed. First, before putting any fluid into or creating any debris in the mouth, make sure the seal of the cuff of the endotracheal tube is adequate. Even if anesthesia is being maintained by injectable agents, an ET tube should be in place. It could be absolutely disastrous if an animal aspirated (inhaled) bacteria and debris from a dental prophy. With the cough reflex eliminated by anesthesia, these would lodge deep in the lungs and at the very least cause pneumonia.

The best way to check the seal of the ET tube is with a pressure manometer connected to the anesthesia bag. Enough air should be injected into the cuff reservoir to maintain a seal when the gas reservoir bag is squeezed (with the exhaust, or "pop-off," valve closed) to measure 15 mm Hg. The ET tube should leak at 20 mm Hg. Putting too much air in causes the cuff to overinflate, which can cause necrosis in the tracheal lining. If there is not a manometer available, the reservoir should be filled just until it is full but softly spongy or until the cuff does not leak as the bag (with closed exhaust valve) is squeezed no harder than you would squeeze a barely ripe tomato to avoid bursting it.

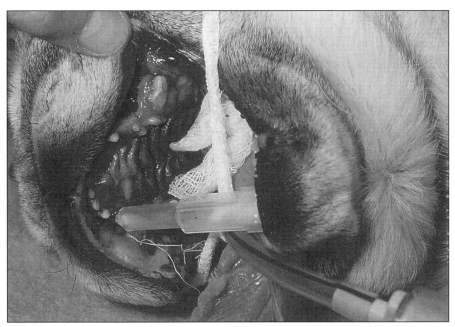

Figure 5-3

The animal is prepared for the prophy with endotracheal intubation and gauze in the pharynx to avoid liquid flowing into the larynx and trachea. A tape over the forehead will remind whoever is extubating to remove the gauze.

It is very important to *open* the exhaust valve after testing the cuff, or the animal eventually will be unable to exhale (or, therefore, breathe) because the oxygen and gas being supplied by the machine completely fills the bag.

If an anesthesia gas odor arises during the procedure, the cuff is allowing leakage. This is often due to relaxation of the laryngeal muscles, and the cuff should be reinflated until leakage ceases. Another possibility, of course, is that the cuff leaks or that the tube has pulled out of the trachea.

A gauze sponge or paper towel stuffed in the back of the mouth to keep debris from accumulating between the mouth and ET tube cuff will further protect the larynx, trachea, and lungs (Fig. 5-3). Again, it is most important to remove these at the end of the procedure.

Making sure that there is adequate ophthalmic ointment in the eyes will keep the corneas from drying and prevent infection by aerosolized bacteria. Some people place a towel over the face and eyes to prevent exposure of the eyes to bacteria (Fig. 5-4). Towels will also protect the eyes from damage from curing lights that are used for some restoratives ("fillings").

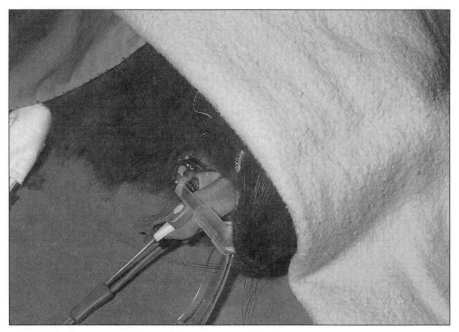

Figure 5-4

A towel over the eyes protects them from the intense glare of the exam light and bacterial scatter.

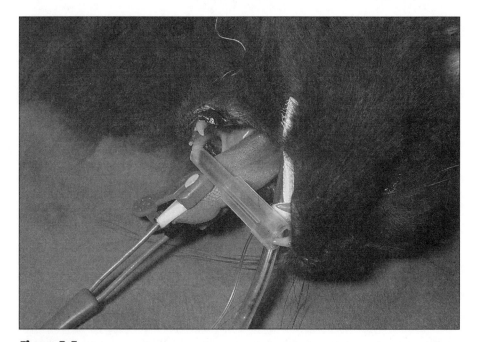

Figure 5-5

A mouth prop made from a plastic catheter container or small syringe barrel costs nothing and can be discarded after one use.

Propping the mouth open greatly facilitates access to all the teeth. The typical commercial mouth gag is a metal **C**-shaped device that has holes on the ends of the arms in which to insert the crowns of the teeth (usually opposing canines), after which the gag is opened wide. These metal holes should be lined with a plastic or rubber material. If they have no resilient lining material, they should not be used because there is a possibility that they can chip or fracture off the teeth. Metal **C**-shaped mouth gags, even if properly lined, could also break teeth if the animal should become light (begin to recover consciousness) and start thrashing around.

An alternative to the metal gags is a simple cylinder of plastic. It could be a cut-off barrel of a syringe, the syringe case in which some syringes come packaged for sterility, or the narrower cases in which some sterile catheters are packaged (Fig. 5-5). We use mostly the catheter cases and do not recycle them after a single use, but these probably could be sanitized and disinfected. One advantage of the plastic, besides not breaking teeth, is that they can be custom trimmed to length for each animal. A disadvantage is that the body of the prop does not stay outside of the mouth, like the **C**-shaped gag. Whichever type of mouth prop is used, it should be on the side toward the table so that you can get into the mouth as freely as possible.

Covering the animal with a blanket or towel, and providing a warm waterblanket between it and the metal table will greatly reduce the chilling that occurs during anesthesia (Fig. 5-6).

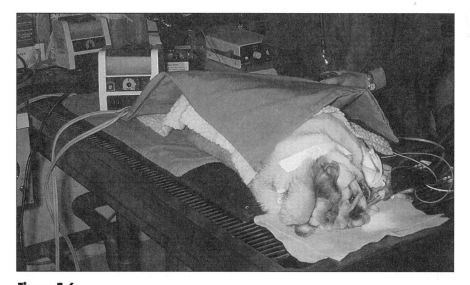

Figure 5-6
The water used in the prophy contributes to the loss of body heat due to anesthesia. Body heat is conserved by a heated waterblanket and by covering the animal's body.

To avoid turning the animal excessively, the prophy is performed from step 1 through 6 (see the following) on one side at a time. The outside of the "up" side of the cheek teeth and the inside of the "down" side are cleaned before the animal is turned over. Half the incisors can be cleaned the same way.

Step 1: Removing Thick Dental Calculus

Some animals accumulate dental calculus to an extraordinary degree. Calculus can be several millimeters thick, especially on the upper fourth premolar near the parotid salivary duct. Happily, this thick crust of calculus is very easy to remove.

To crack off the thick calculus quickly and efficiently, a forceps (either a calculus forceps or an extraction forceps) is simply placed around the tooth with the jaws of the forceps engaging just below the gingiva and squeezed (Fig. 5-7). The calculus will crack off satisfyingly. In many cases, the calculus comes off so thoroughly with the forceps that little more needs to be done to clean the crown. Thin layers of calculus usually do not respond well to the forceps, and these must be taken care of with a scaler. Do not become neurotic about getting every piece of calculus off with the forceps. This is what the ultrasonic and hand scalers are for.

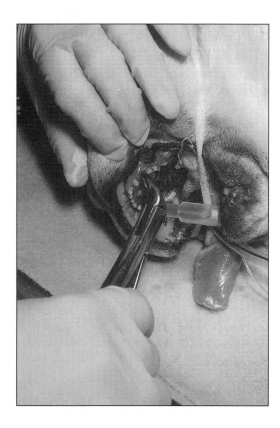

Figure 5-7

A pair of extraction or calculus forceps can be used to crack off thick calculus before scaling.

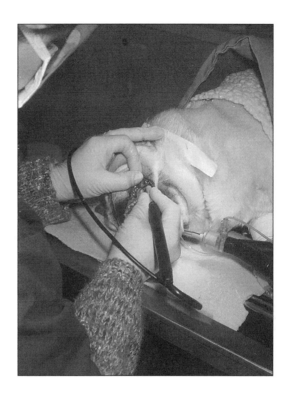

Figure 5-8

The ultrasonic scaler tip must always be cooled by a mist of water.

Step 2: Power Scaling

The entire purpose of a power scaler is to remove calculus quickly. There are three basic power scaler types, ultrasonic, sonic, and rotating metal bur, and their advantages and disadvantages are discussed in Chapter 2. Movement or vibration of the scaler head knocks the calculus off without having to move your hand a lot. The most important thing to remember when using power scalers is that heat is generated with the movement of the scaler. Teeth contain live tissue, and excessive heat applied to that tissue can kill it.

Try this test with an ultrasonic or sonic scaler: Turn on the scaler, apply the tip to a fingernail, and see how many seconds it takes before you feel the burning sensation. It is generally less than 10 seconds. Since the dentinal insulation is thicker than a fingernail, it is safe to assume that a tooth can take 10 seconds of this heat without damage to the pulp. You should use the rule that 10 seconds is the maximum amount of time to spend on any one tooth at any one continuous application. You can always return to an especially dirty large tooth after cleaning one or more others. Rinsing with cold water would also cool the tooth between assaults by the scaler.

Scalers must *always* be water cooled (Fig. 5-8). If water is not flowing when the scaler is on, something is amiss, and it should not touch an animal's mouth. In most scalers, the spray should be adjusted until it fans into a fine mist when it strikes the scaler tip. If the stream of water does not strike the tip, its aperture or the scaler tip has been bent or is maladjusted.

It is also very important to realize that power scalers, whatever type they are, have the potential to damage the surface of the tooth. They should never be passed over every square millimeter of a tooth whether or not there is visible or palpatable calculus covering it. In other words, scaling a tooth is *not* like washing a dirty floor, in which you do every square inch whether there is visible dirt or not. Every time that a scaler touches the tooth, there are at least microscopic (or even visible) scratches in the surface. These tiny surface irregularities allow plaque to attach more readily, and that is why you *always* follow scaling with polishing, to make the surface smooth again.

This abrading action of power scalers is the reason that ultrasonic scalers are seldom used in human dentistry for routine prophies. Over the years, the enamel in human teeth would be (or was, when power scalers were new and many dentists were using them) worn away with annual cleanings. The reason that we can get away with using power scalers in animal dentistry is that the life spans of small animals, who have roughly the same thickness of enamel as humans, are so much shorter than our own.

The particular scaler tip that you use determines how you scale the teeth. With a pointed scaler tip, it can be very gently passed under the gum line, and then visible calculus removed from the rest of the tooth. There is a potential for damage to gingival attachments if a scaler is used too roughly subgingivally, but the advantage is that it will remove most of the calculus on the tooth, and you will not have to spend extensive time hand curetting. The chisel-shaped tip is very useful for pushing calculus off of the teeth in broad swatches and is good for large (dog) teeth. Chisel tips often arrive from the manufacturer with very sharp edges, which can damage the tooth surface by pounding on it. These should be subtly rounded on a sharpening stone before use.

A sharp, pointed ultrasonic scaling tip can be used to engrave metal (although it's not recommended if you want to keep that expensive tip very long). The lesson here is *not* to hold the point against the tooth like a pencil because it could quickly cut through enamel. The way this instrument should be used is to lay the side against the tooth, passing the point under the gum line if desired. Used in this fashion it will remove large areas of calculus rapidly, like the chisel tip. In developmental grooves or other concave surfaces, you should use a hand instrument.

Rotating-metal calculus-removing devices (e.g., the Rotoburr) are falling out of favor in veterinary medicine because they can cause so much damage to the surface of the tooth unless very carefully used. These should never be pushed

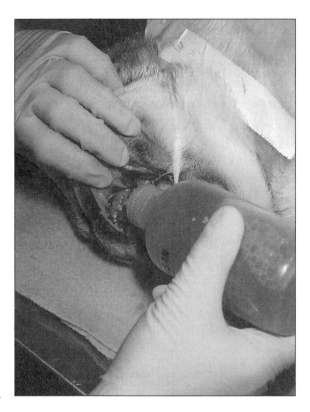

Figure 5-9

A disinfectant rinse before beginning the ultrasonic scaling will greatly decrease the live bacteria aerosolized.

with force against the tooth, but then neither should sonic or ultrasonic tips. If it takes force on the instrument to remove calculus, you have done a poor job of crushing the calculus in step 1.

Before using the power scaler, the operator should rinse the teeth with an oral disinfectant (Fig. 5-9). This will kill many bacteria on contact and reportedly reduce the live bacterial aerosolization about 90 percent. Chlorhexidine gluconate or diacetate at a 0.1 or 0.2 percent concentration is very efficacious. Chlorhexidine gluconate is available from several vendors as an oral disinfectant, which is very effective but is also fairly expensive as compared with diacetate. Chlorhexidine diacetate is available widely and much more inexpensively as a 2 percent concentration of a general disinfectant (Nolvasan). It can easily be diluted to the proper concentration with one part 2 percent solution to nine parts water and stored indefinitely without losing its potency.

Other choices of disinfectants include organic iodine (e.g., Betadine solution) and sanguinaria extract (Viadent mouthwash), but both of these can stain as they are aerosolized. However, they can be useful as an oral rinse after the prophy to cut down on bacteria that can cause local inflammation in the gingiva.

The power scaler handpieces should be held essentially the same as hand instruments to minimize stress to hand and arm and to maintain the fine control of the instrument (see below).

Step 3: Hand Instrumentation

Seldom, except in the case of very mild calculus and no attachment loss, is a prophy adequate with power scalers alone. The only way to check the adequacy of the scaling is with a hand instrument, which usually is a curette but occasionally is a periodontal probe.

Before power scalers were invented, all dental cleanings were performed with a variety of scalers and curettes. In human dentistry, these became so specialized that an instrument might be used on only one tooth or one type of tooth or a particular face of a particular tooth. Dental hygienists still use a wide variety of hand instruments. In general, however, fewer are needed for veterinary dentistry. The reasons are (1) animals' mouths can be opened wider (in general) for better visibility, (2) animals are anesthetized so they can be manipulated for access and visualization, and (3) the bulk of the calculus removal is done with the power scaler.

Most hand instruments used in veterinary dentistry are the same as those used in human dentistry except for one notable exception. This instrument is often sold as simply a "scaler" in veterinary supply houses or groomers' catalogs. It is essentially an enlarged dental hoe, and it is usually double ended so that the two ends can be mirror images of each other (each end has a fairly blunt and a fairly sharp edge). Its flat working face is about 3 mm wide and can clean off a wide path of dental calculus fairly rapidly. Regrettably, some animal hospitals have only this instrument in their dental equipment. Although it can be useful, it is very limited in its application other than removing large areas of calculus on the crowns (Fig. 5-10). As a scaler it should never be used subgingivally (under the gum line). Many veterinary dentists are contemptuous of this instrument, probably because it represents a period when small animal periodontics was nonexistent.

Scalers and curettes differ mainly in the shapes of their cross sections and tips of their working ends (see Chap. 2). A scaler should be used only on the crown of the tooth, mainly because its tip is sharply pointed and if used subgingivally could tear soft tissue. If viewed in cross section, a scaler is triangular. It has a flat face to scrape off calculus and an angle on the backside, unlike the rounded backside of the curette. The angle is much stronger mechanically, and a scaler can be used with much more force before breaking. Because a curette has a rounded end and backside, it can be safely used subgingivally. It can also be used on the crown, but because it is more delicate than the scaler, it tends to break more readily and is gen-

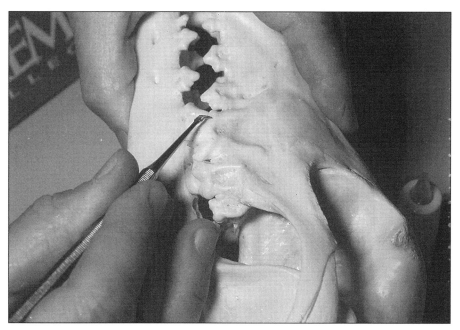

Figure 5-10
A flat scaler such as this will remove broad swatches of calculus on the crowns.

erally a little more expensive. The message here is that you should avoid using curettes as scalers.

The superficial reason for doing a dental prophy is to clean the teeth so that the crowns are white, shiny, and lacking calculus and plaque on the surface. This will please the client, but you know that cleaning the area under and near the gingival margin is critical to stopping the progression of periodontal disease. Any calculus remaining on the crowns after power scaling must be removed not only for aesthetic reasons but also because it can act as a nidus, or seed area, for further calculus.

The most obvious areas that need hand scaling are the developmental grooves and fissures of the teeth. The most notable of these are the notch in the upper fourth premolar and the angle formed by the cingulum of an upper incisor (the shelf at the back of the tooth on which the lower incisor rests).

Other areas that commonly retain calculus are the interproximal areas (spaces between teeth). These are often not a problem unless some periodontal attachment loss has occurred. Often these are too narrow for scalers and must be cleaned with a curette. The most common areas with interproximal calculus in dogs (it seldom occurs in cats because of the anatomy of their teeth) are between incisors, the upper fourth premolar and first molar, the lower first molar and the fourth premolar, and lower first and second molars. These areas are most subject to pocket formation because of the tendency for plaque, and then calculus, to form there.

All hand instruments—the scaler, the hoe (a type of scaler), and the curette—are designed to snap off calculus when their sharp edges are pulled across the surface of teeth. The sharpness of the edge is critical: without a sharp edge the scaler requires more force to pop off calculus, or the instrument simply glides over the calculus and actually burnishes its surface so that it is even harder to make the instrument's edge take hold. The problems with applying more force are that it is more fatiguing for the operator and the instrument will tend to scratch grooves into the tooth surface. (See Chap. 2 for sharpening techniques and recommendations.)

Operator fatigue is a very important consideration. Improper technique can lead to repetitive motion injuries of the wrist or hand. The proper way to use hand instruments is to hold them in a modified pen grip, with the ring and little fingers acting as a balance point so that the other fingers and the thumb can place the instrument in the precise position to begin the stroke. The stroke is then made with a rotation of the shoulder with the lower joints more or less fixed. The absolutely worst thing you can do is use the wrist to make the stroke. The inflammation that can result from repetitive motion injury to the wrist (carpal tunnel syndrome) can be completely debilitating.

There is a greater tendency to injury when using the curette than the scaler. This is because, when used traditionally, the working surface of a curette is placed into a pocket to its bottom, rotated upward to engage the edge, and then pulled out of the pocket. Many people will combine the rotation and pull and do it all with the wrist. One way to avoid this is to place the curette under the gum line with the tip, rather than the rounded edge, facing toward the soft tissue and then to pull as if it were a scaler. This must be done gently to avoid injuring soft tissues, and the tip should be rounded and blunt. (Repeated sharpenings may leave a curette tip pointed rather than rounded.) I feel that a curette used in this fashion is the best way to ensure that no subgingival calculus remains on the teeth. If any rough areas are palpated, they can just be pulled off as the curette contacts them.

Root planing is the term used when normal gingival attachment has been lost and roots must be cleaned of calculus and debris. The calculus that is buried under the gingiva tends to contain bacteria associated with colonization of necrotic tissues; these bacteria tend to produce black or very dark pigments. The dark pigments actually aid in determining whether the root dentin is clean or not. Basically, the root is cleaned until no dark areas or rough patches remain. Sometimes root surfaces are innately rough, and sometimes bacterial action can cause pits and erosions in the dentinal or cementum surfaces. Part of root planing is to restore the smoothness of the root surface so that the gingiva can attach firmly to it. This attachment will not be as tight as to bone, but it can never occur if the dentinal surface is rough.

There are ultrasonic scalers that have very fine tips that are advertised to clean deep pockets. They have the advantage of a constant lavage of water or disinfectant during root cleaning, which flushes debris out of the pockets as they work. Also, they are reputed to cause less damage to the root dentin than a curette. In older humans who have had root planing repeatedly over the years, the neck of the tooth (where the crown meets dentin) is often noticeably narrowed because of the dentin having been scraped away. Usually this is not as much of an issue in animals, but exposed root dentin can suffer considerable attrition with even a single root planing.

Gingival pockets or pseudopockets (a true pocket is formed by a loss of gingival or bony attachment, and a pseudopocket is formed by an overgrowth of gingiva across the tooth surface) must be less than 6 mm deep. Otherwise they will require surgery to adequately clean, either by surgically lifting a mucogingival flap so that the tooth surface can be visualized and cleaned or by amputating extra gingiva at the margin. Any time a pocket exceeds the normal depth of the dental sulcus (4 mm in dogs and 1 mm in cats) and root is exposed, root planing is performed in the process of cleaning the tooth. It is noted on the dental chart as "closed root planing" (RPC) if the depth is under 6 mm and "open root planing" if a surgical flap is used. In most states the practice legislation require the veterinarian to do any oral surgery. The technician's job is to alert the veterinarian to the depths of pockets so that he or she may do the required surgical intervention (see Chap. 9 for information on periodontal surgery).

Step 4: Polishing

Scaling teeth, especially with power scalers, *must* be followed by polishing (Fig. 5-11). As teeth are cleaned, the instruments leave microscopic scratches in the enamel. After enamel has been roughened, plaque adheres more readily. A typical complaint of owners whose pets' teeth had been cleaned for the first time, but not adequately polished, is that a month later their teeth were dirtier than ever.

The polisher, like the scaler, has the potential to harm the tooth pulp with excess heat. To understand how rapidly heat can build up with the polisher, fill the prophy cup with polish, apply it to a fingernail, and start the polisher. Within a few seconds it will be too hot to bear, similar to an ultrasonic scaler. The 10-second rule applies here as well. If a tooth is too big to adequately polish in 10 seconds, you must leave it and come back to it later.

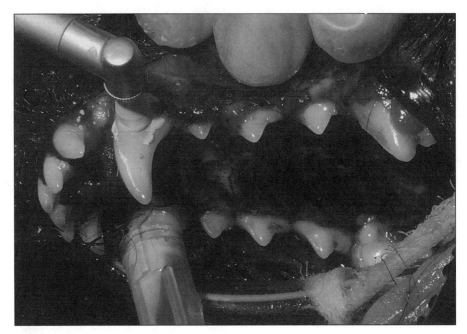

Figure 5-11
To remove microscopic scratches created by the ultrasonic scaler, polishing should always follow ultrasonic scaling.

Like other instruments, the polisher is held in a modified pen grasp. Unlike the scaler, it is important to polish the entire surface of the tooth, even where calculus did not occur. This will serve two purposes. One is that it will remove any soft plaque that may be remaining on the teeth. The other is that the paste is often colored and there is also usually some blood that will mix with the paste; these will stain any light-colored calculus that is left on the tooth. Sometimes calculus is essentially tooth colored and hard to see when you are scaling. You can then scale these areas clean.

The polisher should be passed smoothly over the surface of the tooth rather than moving it rapidly back and forth. It is rotating, so jiggling it around serves no purpose other than possibly missing parts of the tooth. The prophy cup should be pressed against the tooth until the edges flare, and these edges should be passed under the gingival margin to polish subgingivally.

Some people prefer to fill the prophy cup with prophy paste, and others like to apply the paste to the teeth before beginning. Either way works; applying paste first to the teeth may use more paste, but it ensures that adequate paste is on each tooth. If paste is applied with the prophy cup, the simplest way to fill the cup is to turn on the polisher and dip it into the paste; it will burrow into the paste and dig out a portion of it. One of the problems with filling the cup as needed is that it can run out of paste if you are not attentive, in which case you are not polishing but just heating up the tooth. You have to dip the prophy cup into the paste reservoir for virtually every tooth when polishing a large dog's teeth. Another problem (easily remedied) is that a full cup will splatter all over the room if the polisher is accelerated without being against a tooth. If your polisher does not have a foot pedal for on/off and speed, you will have to use the technique with paste on the teeth.

Speed of the polisher and the amount of time spent on each tooth are a concern because of the potential for thermal damage or for inadequately polishing the teeth and leaving them rough. A beginner should keep the polisher at slow speed and move slowly and deliberately over the tooth. Generally about four or five revolutions of the cup are adequate to polish the tooth surface in one area, and when you go slowly, you can count them. As you gain skill, you can increase the speed of the polisher and, correspondingly, the speed over the surface of the teeth. Experts can essentially use the polisher at full speed, which increases the efficiency of the prophy.

After you finish polishing the teeth, they should be thoroughly rinsed. This will allow you to admire what a good job you did or to see any areas that were missed. If you are satisfied with the job, a final rinse with a disinfectant solution helps control bacteria locally; you should massage the disinfectant into the gingival sulci with fingers or gauze or irrigate the sulci with a blunt-tipped needle or canula.

Occasionally you might want to test your work with a disclosing solution. Disclosing solutions come in different colors, usually red or blue. They are dyes that readily bind to plaque and calculus. They can be applied to apparently clean teeth; after rinsing, any color that remains indicates where the teeth have not been cleaned adequately.

Step 5: Dental Probing and Charting

The instrument that is most valuable for diagnosis of dental and periodontal disease is the simple periodontal probe/dental explorer (one instrument, two ends). In human dentistry, the sharp-pointed dental explorer is most often used to feel indentations caused by "cavities" (caries); in veterinary dentistry, it is most likely to be used on dogs and cats to palpate the pulp chamber in open fractures of teeth or to feel the sharp edges of resorptive lesions in cats.

The small blunt end of the periodontal probe is not only useful but necessary to enter and measure dental sulci or pockets (Fig. 5-12). The use of the periodontal probe is very simple. The probe, parallel to the long axis of the tooth, is "walked" gently inside the dental sulcus to its bottom. At least four readings must be made around the circumference of the tooth, but in fact it

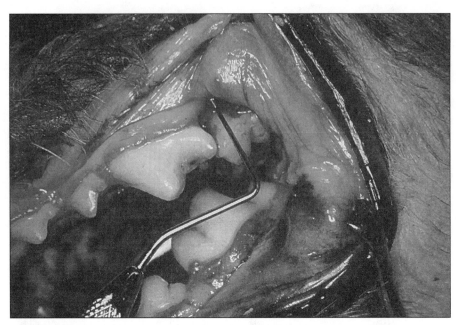

Figure 5-12

The periodontal probe is the most valuable diagnostic tool available to the technician. X rays simply confirm palpation of periodontal pockets and attachment loss.

is usually a continuous palpation so that any areas of loss can be felt. Abnormal depths must be noted on the chart, as well as other abnormalities and therapies. Dental charting is such an important subject and is complex enough that it has its own chapter (Chap. 7).

Step 6: Dental Extractions and Other Surgery

As mentioned above, surgery (dental extractions are considered surgery) is the purview of the veterinarian. The technician indicates teeth that may need extracting. For instance, a tooth for which attached gingiva is completely lacking has no more protection against oral bacteria and is almost certainly doomed. Heroic periodontal surgery could only be performed if adequate attached gingiva is available for a graft. Almost any tooth except lower incisors that shows any mobility is similarly doomed; however, the final decision for extraction must be the veterinarian's. A discussion of exodontic techniques is included in Chapter 8.

If extractions will be performed, local anesthesia can provide postoperative pain relief that is quite profound. It can also decrease the amount of general anesthetic needed for extractions. Local anesthesia for dental extractions is covered in Chapter 6.

Step 7: Animal Recovery, Cleanup, and Prep for Next Case

Before the animal is allowed to recover from anesthesia, its mouth should be thoroughly inspected for blood, water, or other debris that must be removed, particularly in the back of the mouth (the pharyngeal area). Any paper towels or gauze sponges that had been placed to protect the larynx must be removed as well. Gauze and towels could suffocate an animal once the endotracheal tube is removed. Any foreign material left in the pharynx has the potential to be aspirated (breathed into the lungs) before the cough reflex is recovered after anesthesia.

This is also the time to wash blood, prophy paste, and mucus off the animal's face, neck, and shoulders. If blood has been spilled on hair at the catheter site, this should be washed as well. All of this is easier to take care of while the animal is asleep. To prevent unnecessary chilling, the animal should be toweled off as much as possible and placed in a heated cage for recovery, if one is available.

After the animal is extubated and "cage safe," attention can be given to cleanup and preparation for the next prophy, whether it is to follow immediately or not.

Blood, mucus, and other visible soil must be removed from all surfaces and dental instruments, including power instruments, as a first step. Then they can be disinfected and sterilized. Dull instruments should be sharpened after disinfection so that the sharpening stone is not contaminated. See Chapter 2 for specifics of the disinfection/sterilization process. Tables, counters, and positioning equipment are usually wiped down with a disinfecting spray, which is left on the surface for residual effect (not rinsed off afterward). Some veterinary practices reuse prophy cups; these need to be inspected for defects, washed, and placed in a disinfecting solution. They should not be left on the polisher for the next patient.

The final step is to turn off dental equipment after all dental procedures are finished for the day. If a compressor is used, any leaks will result in shortening its effective lifetime of service if it is left on constantly. If a compressed gas source, such as nitrogen, is used for the "air-powered" equipment, leaving it on will mean more frequent replacement of gas bottles. Mechanical scalers that are powered by electricity utilize very little when not in use, but not turning them off is sloppy technique. At the end of the day, no electric device should still have power on; this is only a normal fire precaution.

Anesthesia, Analgesia, and Postsurgical Support

The vast majority of dental patients are older animals because the majority of the procedures are dental prophies, which typically are not performed until cats or dogs are age 3 or 4. Some dental patients are ancient (our oldest dog was 23 and oldest cat was 24). Many have age-related diseases that could complicate anesthesia. In most animal hospitals the technician conducts most, if not all, the anesthesia procedures.

PREANESTHESIA SCREENING

For all animals over the age of 4 years, blood should be drawn for screening. A complete blood count will indicate whether the animal has any of several conditions that could make anesthesia more of a risk. A low packed cell volume, or PCV, indicates anemia, or a decreased number of red blood cells. Red blood cells, or RBCs, carry oxygen and carbon monoxide between the lungs and the rest of the body. If RBCs are low, they cannot do this as effectively, and the rest of the body can become oxygen starved and carbon dioxide saturated. Since all tissues need oxygen to live, this is a serious problem because respiration is depressed during anesthesia. This is the main reason that we use straight oxygen rather than room air as the carrier for the anesthesia gas; straight oxygen makes up for the respiratory depression by providing more oxygen in each breath.

There are many conditions that can cause anemia, but essentially they fall into two categories: blood loss or lack of production of blood cells. Conditions like trauma, bleeding from the intestinal tract, or autoimmune destruction of red blood cells can account for loss, and drug- or cancer-induced bone marrow depression can cause decreased production. Anemia from a chronic disease such as periodontitis can cause a usually mild anemia via bone marrow depression. If an animal is anemic, the veterinarian should investigate the cause and compare the risks with the benefits.

High or low numbers of white blood cells (WBCs) indicate the animal's general health. Large numbers of neutrophils, especially if they show signs of toxicity or immaturity, most likely indicate a severe infection. The infection may be periodontitis, but this condition often exists without causing increases in circulating neutrophils. High numbers of eosinophils and basophils indicate an allergy or parasitism. If the animal has heartworms, the heart could be severely compromised, which is not a good thing combined with the cardiovascular depression that accompanies virtually all general anesthetics. Very low numbers of lymphocytes may indicate stress as the blood was taken (common with cats) or the onset of a viral disease. Any change in cellular morphology (i.e., how the cells look) may indicate disease. Again, the important thing is that a disease condition is known and considered when deciding whether or not to proceed with anesthesia.

High plasma protein may indicate high immunoglobulins (circulating antibodies) because of an allergy, parasitism, or chronic infection. Low plasma protein probably means the liver is not producing albumin, the main protein in the blood, or albumin is being lost, as by chronic gastrointestinal disease. Since many drugs are ordinarily "protein bound" in the circulation, a lack of protein to bind to will change the effect on the body; the tendency is that too much of the drugs will be made available to the body and cause an overdose. Underlying liver disease causing low protein in the blood also has serious potential complications regarding the liver being able to handle the drugs.

The blood chemistries required for anesthesia are those that would indicate compromise in the major drug-metabolizing organs, the liver and kidney. A minimum of one liver enzyme (usually alk phos—alkaline phosphatase—or SGOT) will show whether there is an active problem with the liver. The kidneys can be assessed through BUN (blood urea nitrogen) and creatinine levels. Most older dogs and cats have slightly elevated levels of liver enzymes and/or BUN, but extremely high levels may preclude anesthesia.

A good physical exam is a must before anesthesia (Fig. 6-1). Although an increased temperature may result strictly from excitement, it could indicate an emerging generalized infection. The heart rate is also responsive to stress or excitement, but if it is exceptionally high, it could indicate a hyperthyroid or cardiomyopathic cat, for instance. The lungs and heart should always be auscultated; abnormally harsh lung sounds, or rales that sound like whistles as the animal breathes, could be signs of pneumonia or backup of fluid in the lungs due to a weak heart. Heart murmurs are signs that the heart is not working to normal capacity. In the final analysis it is the veterinarian's decision to proceed with anesthesia, but as the technician, you may be asked to do the preanesthesia physical (as often happens). You should bring all abnormalities to the veterinarian's attention.

This is not to say that even a serious condition should necessarily cancel anesthesia. A cat or dog with an enlarged heart as well as severe periodontitis or an abscessing tooth should not be subject to the constant showers of bacteria that these conditions create. Any heart condition in which normal function is compromised is more subject to infection by the constantly circulating oral bacteria, and the animal will do better in the long run if its mouth is allowed to heal. Also, a dog or cat with diabetes is more susceptible to infections like periodontitis, and the infection may keep the animal from being regulated to a normal blood glucose by its insulin injections. Therefore, even though anesthesia may

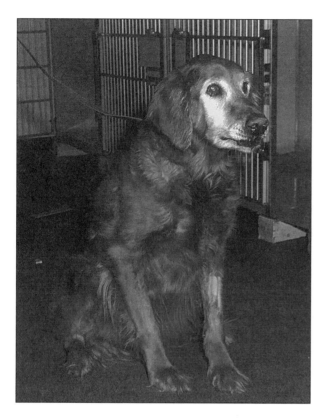

Figure 6-1

Because many of our dental patients are old animals with the possibility of age-related conditions, it is important to have a good physical exam and database before anesthetizing them.

cause transient abnormal blood glucose levels, the animal is better off relative to its disease as well as its comfort level after the infection is dealt with.

ANESTHESIA MEDICATIONS

Antibiotics need to be at therapeutic blood levels at the time of the dental prophy (Fig. 6-2). The easiest and most certain method for this is to give the antibiotic intravenously (IV) after the animal is anesthetized but before beginning the prophy. Ampicillin and cephalexin are very useful for IV administration. As an alternative, antibiotics can be administered subcutaneously or intramuscularly while the animal is awaiting anesthesia; generally this must be done at least an hour before anesthesia. Antibiotics also may be sent home with the owner at a previous visit with instructions for administration. In a filthy mouth it will be obvious when the animal returns if the owner has complied with antibiotic administration because the inflammation, and probably the odor, will be greatly decreased. If there is any doubt whether the owner has been getting oral antibiotics into the animal, the animal should be given a similar drug by injection.

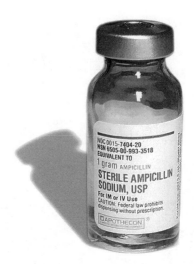

Figure 6-2

During the prophy, support with antibiotics is desirable to avoid seeding organs with bacteria released into the bloodstream.

In general the trend in dental anesthesia is to use drugs that antagonize the health of the older patient as little as possible. This means the use of drugs that can be turned off or reversed if the animal gets into trouble under anesthesia. In fact what this boils down to is an "ideal" recipe that applies for most animals, which is outlined below.

The easiest choice of drug is the gas anesthetic. There is only one, isoflurane, that does not require the body to break it down (metabolize it) in some way (Fig. 6-3). The animal is maintained asleep by the isoflurane as soon as levels absorbed through the lungs are high enough in the bloodstream to cause unconsciousness. As soon as the anesthetic is no longer delivered to the lungs, the animal "blows off" the gas with each breath until it wakes up; the animal continues to release the gas until it is totally out of its system. Some practices induce and maintain animals with isoflurane alone. This is particularly useful for small animals like cats or small dogs that can be "boxed down" in an anesthesia chamber or very quiet dogs that can be "masked down" with isoflurane. Note that this gas is fairly expensive, however, and animals that are apparently healthy may not require this precaution.

Most animals are given a preanesthetic that prepares them for some of the depressive effects of general anesthesia. Atropine and glycopyrrolate are drugs that antagonize parasympathetic nerves. They are necessary because the parasympathetic nervous system maintains functions that are good for normal everyday life: a nice, slow heart rate, the production of saliva and other respiratory secretions, and the muscular movement of the gut when digesting foodstuff. The saliva, respiratory secretions produced by the lungs and airways, and slow heart rate are contraindicated in an animal under anesthesia. In this state, the animal does not swallow or cough and may have a depressed heart rate from the anesthesia.

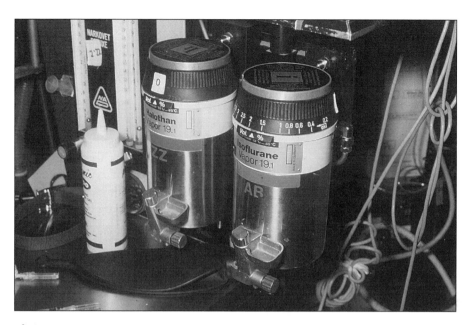

Figure 6-3
Isoflurane is a popular and effective gas anesthetic.

The vagus nerve is the parasympathetic nerve to the heart. "Vagus tone," or the effect of stimulation of this nerve, is demonstrated by a slow heart rate with sinus arrhythmia. (In sinus arrhythmia the heart rate slows when the animal takes a breath because there is pressure on the vagus nerve from the inflated lungs; the rate speeds up when the animal breathes out.) Administration of atropine or glycopyrrolate will speed up the heart to a steady rhythm that does not respond to breathing, usually within about 10 minutes if the drug is given subcutaneously. These two drugs are generally considered benign, although they do require some metabolism by the liver. Each should be administered at a sufficient time before general anesthesia to take full effect. Note that the effective period of each may be as little as 20 minutes, so if the heart rate slows during anesthesia, the drug may need to be redosed.

There are two basic reasons for other preanesthetic agents. One reason is sedation, and the other is analgesia (pain relief). Both have enhancing effects for the gas anesthesia. Sedation increases the nonresponsiveness of general anesthesia, and analgesia allows the animal to be less deeply unconscious but still not respond to painful stimuli.

Sedation aids in the handling of the animal in the induction period when the transition from consciousness to unconsciousness occurs. This can be a frightening experience for an animal, and its instinct is to escape. Reducing anxiety is the main function of sedation in premedication, and when it is effective, it makes the animal amenable to such procedures as placing an IV catheter for induction drugs.

A traditional drug for sedation in dogs and cats is acepromazine, but it is a poor choice for elderly patients. It can cause profoundly low blood pressure because it causes dilation of the blood vessels. The low blood pressure can effectively reduce blood supply to vital organs, the most important of which are the kidneys. Unfortunately, especially in older animals with kidneys that have lost much of their function already, the loss of several thousand more nephrons (the individual units that filter out the wastes and concentrate the urine) due to a decreased blood supply could throw them into kidney failure. Acepromazine also requires liver metabolism, and some animals, because of poor liver function, will stay under its effects for days.

Since there are several reasons we want dental patients to go home the same day they receive anesthetics, we want to avoid drugs that have lasting sedative effects. One reason is that many of these older animals do better at home, where they are not anxious and can get more individualized attention. Also, many hospitals do not have 24-hour care and would have to transfer patients overnight if they were not ready to go home at closing time.

Many older patients will need extractions after their prophies, and pain relief is indicated to supplement anesthesia gas and to help the animal during recovery. Pain control is always most effective if it is given prophylactically. Once pain is felt by the animal, it may cause an increased sensitivity to pain, and a cascade of increasing waves of pain may result. A class of drugs that is helpful for sedation and analgesia for dogs is the opioids. Morphine (Fig. 6-4) and fentanyl are both effective; morphine has the advantage of being inexpensive, but it almost always makes dogs vomit through an effect on the vomiting center of the brain. It also causes smooth muscle contraction and may induce defecation, vomiting, or urination. Fentanyl is more powerful and often a better sedative, but it is shorter acting (with a duration of action of about two hours, as compared with up to four or five hours for morphine). If the desire is for longer-lasting pain relief, the better drug is morphine, but animals getting morphine may be quite "drunk" even several hours after the dental procedure.

All opioids cause cardiac and respiratory depression and so need to be used carefully. Their one big advantage is that an antagonist drug can be administered that will completely reverse the excessive sedative effects. Unfortunately, the antagonist drug can reverse analgesic effects at the same time.

Of course opioids have one great disadvantage: They are class II drugs that have to be kept under lock and key and carefully administered and logged. Failure to do so will get your employer in trouble with the Drug Enforce-

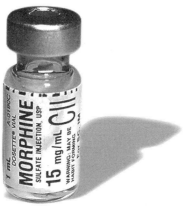

Figure 6-4
Morphine has both analgesic and sedative effects as a premedication. It usually causes an animal to vomit shortly after administration.

ment Administration. But anesthesia, realistically, cannot be performed without controlled drugs.

Cats can be a problem if they do not achieve adequate premedication sedation. They sometimes experience excitement with opioids. Under opioid influence alone they occasionally just do not get sedated enough to handle for induction. To avoid the problem, cats may be induced with an anesthesia chamber without preanesthetic sedation. One of the things that works against you is allowing a cat to become unduly stressed by handling in the induction period. The adrenaline the cat produces can have very negative effects when combined with other drugs such as ketamine or halothane. The most negative effect is the heart stopping, a severe side effect in anyone's opinion. Although the cat will be stressed with an anesthesia chamber, the fact that it is not manually restrained is an advantage. And use of isoflurane precludes the need for the sometimes troublesome halothane and ketamine.

If an animal is not "boxed down" or "masked down," other drugs will have to be given to allow intubation. The usual route is IV because of the desire for speed and the fact that one class of drugs commonly used for induction, the barbiturates, can only be given IV because of severe reactions with tissues if given outside of a vein. Barbiturates at one time were the only class of drugs for anesthesia induction, and sloughing of tissues was a fairly common occurrence, especially when drugs were given by needle directly into the vein in a moving animal.

Only the ultra–short-acting barbiturates (e.g., thiopental) should be used for anesthesia induction if barbiturates are desired, and then only through a catheter that is guaranteed to be in the vein. A barbiturate is given fairly rapidly to effect profound unconsciousness. Unfortunately, as well as allowing intubation, the drug also often causes apnea (cessation of breathing). Another problem that may occur is excitement or struggling; if this happens, additional drug should be rapidly infused, or the animal could hurt itself or personnel. A barbiturate has the peculiarity of having an affinity to fat and rapidly enters fat depots in the body from the bloodstream, after which the fat slowly releases the drug back into the blood where it must be removed and metabolized by the liver. Barbiturates can be highly toxic to dogs that have no fat depots, like sight hounds, because virtually all the drug stays in the blood to cause depression of the brain and poisoning of the liver with excessive drug.

There are no drugs that counteract barbiturates, so the only option is to wait for the effects to wane. In general, the barbiturates may not be a good choice for older dogs: they may be obese and will thereby store large amounts of the drug, which can cause depression for days on end. Thiopental can be used on cats, but there are much better alternatives.

Ketamine, with or without Valium (diazepam), can be used for induction in cats IM (intramuscularly), SC (subcutaneously), or IV. However, rapid administration IV in an excited cat may (rarely) cause the heart to stop. In general ketamine is a safe drug for cats, causing minimal depression of heart rate and breathing. One problem is that many cats have "bad trips" because ketamine is a powerful hallucinogenic drug. Ketamine also must be metabolized by the kidneys in cats (the liver in dogs), and cats with renal (kidney) compromise should not be given the drug. Recently, ketamine has become a controlled drug because of potential for human abuse.

Ketamine and Valium can be given IV to dogs for induction. Ketamine should not be administered to dogs without diazepam because it can cause seizures in dogs. However, with the antiseizure medication Valium, it is quite safe; dogs as well as cats experience a similar lack of depression of heart rate and breathing. Valium also tends to eliminate an effect of ketamine sometimes seen in cats, a rigidity of the limbs (extensor rigidity). This effect results from ketamine-induced interruption of tracts in the brain that modulate muscle tension. Furthermore, Valium tends to "smooth out" the general effects of ketamine hallucinations in cats.

Ketamine and Valium have a tendency to precipitate (become solid, beginning with a slight cloudiness) when mixed and stored together and so should be mixed just before administration. Ketamine and Valium are a favorite induction agent in many practices. The combination is safe for sight hounds, and it will not cause a slough of tissues if administered outside of a vein (an exception may occur if huge amounts are injected).

A drug that is utilized in some practices for induction is very similar to ketamine/diazepam: tiletamine/zolazepam (a.k.a. Telazol). As the names suggest, the components are simply different variations in the same drug classes. Telazol is useful for IM injection for rapidly reducing an aggressive dog to uncon-sciousness, but it is expensive. Essentially it can be used the same as keta-mine/diazepam.

Another drug finding more use in veterinary medicine is propofol. A milky-looking liquid, it is widely used in human medicine either as a constant IV infusion to maintain anesthesia along with a powerful opioid for pain or as a single injection for induction. It is very popular because unconsciousness is rapidly attained and recovery of consciousness occurs very rapidly after the drug is withdrawn.

Veterinary use is usually limited to induction of gas anesthesia. Propofol, unlike barbiturates or ketamine/Valium, should be administered slowly to effect. With fluids flowing, the propofol is injected into the line until a diluted "skim milk" whiteness is achieved. The slower it is given, the less it usually takes to cause unconsciousness. Since this is a very expensive drug, slow administration is a money saver. Also, if it is given rapidly, it almost always causes cessation of breathing, which can be distressing to personnel and make it necessary to intubate quickly and force breaths into the animal. There is seldom any excitement with propofol administration; animals just sink down, asleep. If they are too responsive to intubation, more drug is given.

Propofol seems to be a very effective drug, except that it should never be used alone for painful procedures. An apparently unconscious animal will react violently to pain, even though it will allow intubation and nonpainful manip-ulation. Propofol does require liver metabolism, but it seems fairly benign for most animals, except, perhaps, those in liver failure or with decreased liver function (small liver, blood vessel shunts around the liver, etc.). Preloading with fluids (half an hour's dose) may prevent the transient hypotension that sometimes occurs with IV administration.

Which anesthetic gas to use has already been alluded to. Isoflurane, although it is expensive, has the advantage of rapid induction (with box or mask), quick recovery, and no metabolism by the body. Sevoflurane results in even faster induction and recovery but requires liver metabolism; it is also expen-sive and so is not really an improvement over isoflurane. Many practices still use halothane, which is more cost-effective but results in slower induction and recovery, requires liver metabolism, and can cause arrhythmias (abnor-mal rhythms, such as premature ventricular contractions, or PVCs) when combined with an excited animal's adrenaline or with epinephrine use. The advantage of any anesthetic gas is that once it is turned off it begins to be elim-inated. Monitored judiciously, virtually any anesthetic gas can be safely administered to any but catastrophically ill animals.

ANESTHESIA MONITORING

The one parameter that best indicates an animal's condition and its anesthesia survivability is blood pressure. There are machines used on human patients that automatically measure the systolic and diastolic blood pressure every few minutes through a blood pressure cuff that fills and empties automatically. Most of the time they are quite accurate for medium to large dogs but are expensive.

An alternative is the use of a doppler crystal hooked to a machine that allows you to hear the pulse (Fig. 6-5). You then manually take blood pressure with a cuff and manometer, and the doppler sound tells you when you have reached the pressure that represents the systolic blood pressure (typically you pump the manometer past the place where the sound disappears and then slowly let the pressure out until you hear it again). Essentially you are using the doppler to hear the pulse because it is very difficult with small animals to auscultate the pulse with a stethoscope as is done for humans. Although you cannot get a diastolic blood pressure with a doppler setup, it is much less important than systolic. The systolic tells you the amount of force being used to pump the blood to a limb or tail.

If the blood pressure is adequate to perfuse the periphery, it is generally adequate to perfuse important internal organs like the kidneys and brain. If there is any doubt whether kidney perfusion is adequate (as, for instance, in an animal with

Figure 6-5

Monitoring equipment should be used to assess the animal's condition under anesthesia. This doppler unit measures blood pressure, which is the variable most predictive of survival.

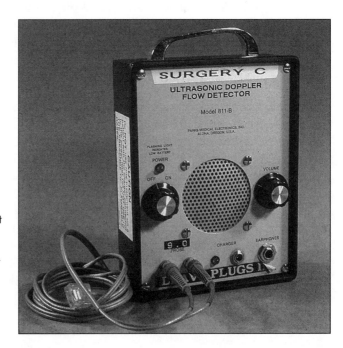

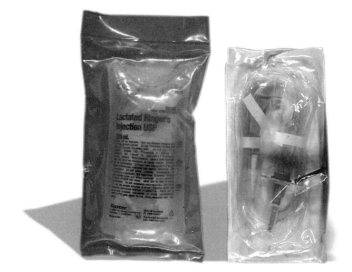

Figure 6-6

Support with IV fluids, with a catheter in place in case life-saving drugs should be needed, is standard for older animal anesthesia.

borderline kidneys), you should give a constant infusion of a drug that specifically increases renal perfusion, such as dopamine or dobutamine.

If blood pressure in the periphery (legs or tail) falls below 70 in a cat or 90 in a dog, the first thing that should be done is to reduce the anesthesia gas. If the animal gets too light (begins to recover consciousness) when the gas is reduced but the pressure is still low, the next thing you should consider doing is to administer fluids in a bolus (a large quantity).

Blood pressure drops when there is less fluid (blood) in the vessels and heart. This can happen with acute blood loss but also may be a problem with an animal whose kidneys cannot concentrate urine or that simply has not had enough water to drink in the past few hours. All older animals should have a catheter and fluids, such as lactated ringer's solution, flowing throughout the anesthesia (Fig. 6-6). The normal rate of infusion of fluids is 10 ml/kg/hour. This means that a 20 kg (44 lb) dog should be receiving 200 ml during an hour's anesthesia. Since in a normal drip set there are 15 drops per ml, you can figure how fast the fluid should drip per second by this formula:

$$\frac{\text{ml needed}}{\text{1 hour}} \times \frac{\text{1 hour}}{\text{60 minutes}} \times \frac{\text{1 minute}}{\text{60 seconds}} \times \frac{\text{15 drops}}{\text{ml}} = \frac{\text{drops}}{\text{second}}$$

The maintenance dose of fluid for the 20 kg (44 lb) dog is 5/6 of a drop per second, or 5 drops in 6 seconds. If you think the animal may not have been drinking adequate water (if, for instance, it has been resting in a cage for four hours waiting for its dental prophy), you can safely give it half an hour's dose of fluid in a bolus and repeat that amount once. (If the animal was noticeably dehydrated before anesthesia, you would calculate how dehydrated and get that amount of fluid to it as soon as possible while the animal was awaiting anesthesia; then you would give it its maintenance dose. However, this situation should not arise for a prophy.) If an animal has a history of PU/PD (polyuria/polydipsia, or urinating all the time because it drinks a lot of water), it should have water available all the time while in the hospital, except while under the influence of anesthesia. If the cause of the PU/PD is borderline kidney function, withholding water will throw the animal into a renal crisis and may well kill it.

If turning down the gas and providing fluid in a bolus do not bring blood pressure up, the animal may need drugs to increase the tone of the peripheral blood vessels and increase the strength of cardiac contractions. The most frequently used drug for this purpose is ephedrine, a stimulant. It can be given as a single dose or as a constant infusion. Infusion pumps that deliver a certain amount of a small quantity of fluid into a fluid line are extremely convenient when constant infusions are indicated. The amount is calculated based on (1) how much fluid an animal needs per hour as determined by its weight and (2) the amount of drug to be added to the fluid line in that time.

Hypertension (high blood pressure) is extremely rare in dogs and cats under anesthesia (it is virtually unheard of). Hypotension (low blood pressure), however, is frequently a problem. The anesthetic drugs, with few exceptions, cause a depression of the blood pressure to a greater or lesser extent. Blood pressure is a very good indicator of anesthesia depth. As the animal gets too deep, blood pressure drops. If you cannot measure blood pressure with a cuff, you should use other sources of information for an animal's depth of anesthesia. One is the strength of the pulse. The feel of the pulse will change with pressure change; it will become less bounding and more feeble as blood pressure falls.

Many practices have invested in pulse oximeter machines (Fig. 6-7). These utilize the passage of light through thin skin to sense the pulsation of blood through capillaries and to read the amount of oxygen in the blood. These show at least that there *is* blood being pumped through peripheral tissues and, if oxygenation stays high, that there is an adequate amount of blood being pumped (which, after all, is what we are trying to determine when we auscultate the pulse). Pulse oximeters are equipped with alarms that tell when a pulse cannot be sensed or when oxygenation has fallen. However, they can be defective, and we are anesthetizing a patient, not a machine.

When you are working on the mouth, you have a wonderful indicator of oxygenation of the tissues right at your fingertips—the tongue, gingiva, and

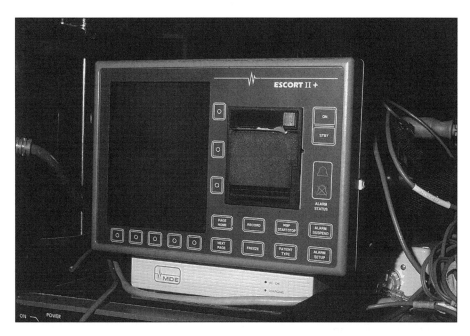

Figure 6-7

The pulse oximeter has become popular in many hospitals. It measures oxygen saturation and heart rate.

mucous membranes. Pink is good; grayish or bluish is bad. Pink means there is lots of oxygen in the blood, and blue means there is a lot of carbon dioxide instead. Gradual blanching, or whitening, of the gingiva and mucous membranes is common if they get dryish. If they *suddenly* blanch, this could signal cardiac asystole (the heart stopped). A pulse can be felt on each side of the underside of the tongue. Periodic monitoring of its strength is another way to assess the animal's condition.

Another machine that indirectly signals that an animal is doing all right is the apnea monitor. This machine has a sensor in a tube that fits between the endotracheal tube and the anesthesia machine's delivery tube(s). Every time the animal takes a breath, the monitor will make a reassuring beep. The monitor is set for a certain number of breaths a minute, and if it doesn't sense them, it sets off an alarm.

You can be well assured that your animal's heart is still beating if it is breathing, but you have no assurance that its kidneys are getting enough blood flow. In the final analysis, good anesthesia can be boiled down to three things: (1) The fewer drugs used, the better, and drugs should be avoided that cannot be withdrawn or reversed or that cause undue negative effects; (2) anesthesia is best kept as light as possible to get the job done; and (3) monitoring should first depend on direct observation of the patient and then on helpful machines. Much of anesthesia is an art, and evaluating the rhythm and flow of it becomes second nature. You should never become complacent about anesthesia, however. The health of these animals is in your hands.

SUGGESTED REGIMES FOR MINIMALLY INVASIVE ANESTHESIA

Dogs: Premed with 0.04 mg/kg atropine and (1) 1 mg/kg morphine sulfate (if anticipating extractions) or (2) 0.01 mg/kg fentanyl (if not expecting extractions); these may be combined in the same syringe to be administered SC. Induce with (1) ketamine 5 to 10 mg/kg and Valium 0.2 mg/kg (give entire dose) or (2) propofol 4 to 6 mg/kg drawn up (give slowly to effect), either one to be administered IV via previously placed catheter. Intubate and maintain on isoflurane.

Cats: Premed with 0.04 mg/kg atropine SC. Box induce with isoflurane and intubate as soon as practical. Maintain on isoflurane. It is easiest to place the catheter after the cat is asleep.

PATIENT POSITIONING AND SUPPORT DURING THE DENTAL PROCEDURE

For almost all dental procedures it is adequate for the animal to be in lateral recumbency. Virtually the only time when the animal must be in dorsal or ventral recumbency rather than on its side is when a full-mouth impression is made.

A dental prophy almost always involves copious amounts of water for the ultrasonic scaler and to rinse the animal's mouth. If some sort of flow table is not available, towels should be changed as soon as they begin to get waterlogged. The head (especially the underside) tends to get very wet, and the evaporation that occurs will chill the animal because a major portion of the blood supply passes through the brain and will be cooled.

Even if the animal is not on a metal table, it will tend to get cold during anesthesia because the brain cannot regulate body heat when the animal is unconscious. At the least an anesthetized animal should have a towel or blanket under it to protect it from the warmth-stealing metal rack; it is much preferable to have a waterblanket (Fig. 6-8) to supply extra heat. Waterblankets are thermostatically controlled so that heated water is passed evenly through them, without the hot spots (often found in electric heating pads) that could cause burns. For very small dogs and cats, a waterbed of unopened fluid bags

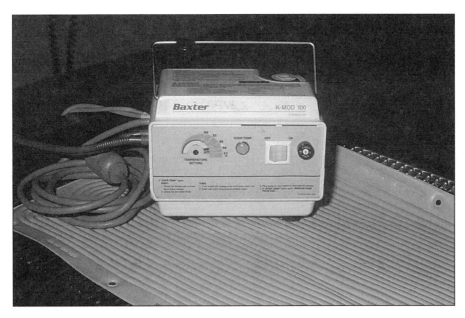

Figure 6-8
The waterblanket supports the body temperature of the patient.

can be rigged. The bags can be heated in an incubator where they are stored or may carefully be heated in a microwave. If you can't hold the bag against the back of your hand, the inside of your wrist, or your cheek for one minute, it is too hot. The importance of keeping the animal warm relates to the metabolism of drugs. The enzymatic reactions that take place in the liver and other organs are affected by temperature. A general rule in chemistry is that a chemical reaction is cut in half for every decrease of 10 degrees Celsius, so you can see that the colder an animal is the less able it will be to overcome the effects of its drugs.

Another aid to keeping an animal warm is to cover it. Even though the dog or cat has a hairy coat to help insulate it against the cold, the blanket will help retain any body heat the animal produces. The smaller the animal, the more heat will be lost because of the increase in surface area relative to the animal's mass. Some people wrap very small animals in plastic bags and tie them at the neck. This not only keeps warmth in but keeps the hair of the body from being wetted.

After the procedure, if the animal has blood or other debris on the hair of its head, you will need to wash it off. This is where a flow table with a warm spray is very handy. The animal should be cleaned and toweled off as thoroughly as possible before being put in the recovery cage.

A variety of small pads and sandbags can be fashioned to allow the head to be lifted off of the table or to stabilize it in a certain position. They should be covered in plastic so that they may be disinfected. For example, a pad may be covered with a plastic wastebasket liner taped together. If a plastic bag cover should get too soiled to wipe off with disinfectant, it can easily be discarded. It is a good idea to provide padding under the face during extractions because the side of the face can incur trauma when pushed against a metal table; several layers of folded-up towel does very well.

When extraction sites are to be sutured or any other oral surgery is to be performed, it is a good idea to have the hairy face toweled out with one or two towels and towel clamps. Without towels, tiny hairs from the dog will pull into the surgery or extraction sites, and it is a nuisance to attempt to keep them out.

A mouth prop of some sort is necessary for many dental procedures. In general, it should be placed between the upper and lower canines on the down side. A prop of plastic tubing, such as a catheter sleeve or (for cats) a needle cover with the end cut off, is safer than the **C**-shaped expanding mouth gags. If however, these gags are used, they should be taken out before animals are turned. These gags should never be used if they lack the rubber liners for inserting teeth into. They just have too much potential for breaking teeth.

Many times it is prudent to stuff gauze into the back of the animal's mouth to minimize the flow of water and debris into the pharynx. The cuff on the endotracheal tube, of course, should always be inflated, but fluid could still enter the larynx. If you put gauze or a towel into the pharynx, *you must remember to remove it*. The last thing you should do in every dental procedure is to inspect the rear of the mouth to assure yourself it is totally clean and to wipe it if it is not. A gauze or towel in the pharynx could suffocate an animal recovering from anesthesia.

ANALGESIA

Although in the past, when pain control was not nearly as sophisticated as it is now, many animals with severe periodontitis seemed in *less* pain just after extractions than they were before, there were also animals that seemed totally miserable. If we were to have teeth extracted, we would expect to have the pain controlled as well as possible, and this is what we should do for our pets.

When we have a tooth drilled or extracted, the dentist administers a local anesthetic in a regional block. A local anesthetic used for human dentistry tends to last for a few hours, in which we drool and chew our lips, tongue, or cheeks. We can catch ourselves before we do drastic damage to the soft tissues, but dogs and cats don't understand that the reason their mouths won't close is because their tongues or lips are between their teeth, and their teeth are sharper than ours. Therefore in animal dentistry we minimize the number of regional blocks we do with local anesthetics.

One of the most difficult of regional blocks is the mandibular nerve, which can be infiltrated where it enters the inside of the angle of the jaw from the inside of the mouth or from underneath the jaw through the skin. However, blocking at this level will affect tongue, lips, and cheek, and the potential for trauma is high, so it is better not to even attempt it.

The infraorbital foramen contains the infraorbital branch of the maxillary nerve, which serves all of the teeth rostral to (in front of) the eye, palate, nose, and upper lips. Usually the upper lips do not get caught in the teeth (unless an upper canine is extracted), so the potential for trauma is low, and a regional block of this nerve will deaden several extraction sites. If the needle is directed into the infraorbital canal, the fourth premolar and molars may be deadened also. The infraorbital canal can be palpated by lifting the lip and feeling for a divot in the bone just in front of the mesial buccal root tip of the upper fourth premolar.

Before injecting any local anesthetic, one should be sure to aspirate the syringe, and if blood comes into the syringe, never inject it. First, it will not block the nerve if it is placed in a vessel, and second, it can have profound effects on the heart. Many preparations of lidocaine contain epinephrine for local analgesia because the epinephrine causes local vasospasm (contraction of the muscles of the vessels) and extends the local effects longer by not allowing the blood to carry it away. Uncontrolled epinephrine, especially if the animal is anesthetized with halothane, could cause serious cardiac arrhythmias, so lidocaine with epinephrine should never be used for local anesthesia in the mouth in this case.

A general procedure for regional blocking is to keep the needle as close to the surface as possible and to inject a small amount to form a "bleb." This can be repeated until the blebs coalesce when blocking the skin. A large bleb over a nerve, for instance, just in front of the infraorbital canal, can serve for a regional block.

Since we may not want to have a regional block, a local block of an alveolus is often the answer (Fig. 6-9). After extracting a tooth, cleaning out granulomatous and necrotic debris, and suturing the extraction site, a small amount of local anesthetic may be injected deep into each root socket. The total amount of local anesthetic that can be safely administered to a dog or cat is approximately 2 mg/kg, and this must be divided between extraction sites if there are several. A combination of bupivacaine and lidocaine with epineph-

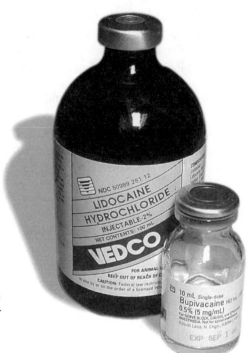

Figure 6-9

Local blocks (instilling local anesthetic directly into extraction sites) and regional blocks of nerve trunks will make patients who have undergone extractions substantially more comfortable for several hours after anesthesia.

rine has proved very effective for hours of pain control when administered intra-alveolarly.

The long-lasting analgesic effects of morphine are discussed earlier in the chapter. This drug is quite effective at keeping pain at bay for several hours. An animal may be redosed with morphine after dental surgery, but it is important that its body temperature be above 100 degrees Fahrenheit before administration. One of the signs of overdosing of morphine is hypothermia (abnormally cold body temperature), another is bradycardia (low heart rate), and a third is oversedation. Morphine should never be given if any of these signs are present. Similarly, fentanyl patches can be applied to the skin to supply a constant amount of the drug until the patch is removed, but the absorption does not reach an effective level in the blood for several hours.

There are other analgesics besides the opioids. The nonsteroidal antiinflammatory drugs (also known as NSAIDs) are quite effective for the soft tissue and bone pain of extractions. An injection of the ibuprofen-like drug ketoprofen can extend pain relief up to 12 hours. As soon as an animal can eat (because the drug can cause gastric upset by eroding the stomach lining), it can get oral aspirin at 10 mg/kg every 12 hours for dogs and every 48 hours for cats (the enzyme that breaks down aspirin in the liver is greatly reduced

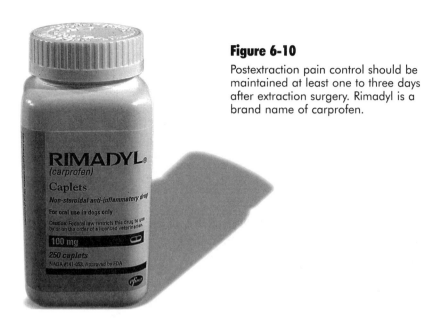

Figure 6-10
Postextraction pain control should be maintained at least one to three days after extraction surgery. Rimadyl is a brand name of carprofen.

in cats). Carprofen has been recommended for older animals for arthritis, and it can be dispensed for postextraction pain as well (Fig. 6-10).

The usual acute period for extraction pain is 24 to 48 hours, and if the pain can be controlled during that time the animal will usually rapidly recover. Note that the NSAIDs, especially aspirin, may cause a decrease in clotting ability, but they have never been a problem in this author's experience. Cats should never be given acetaminophen (Tylenol) because it is toxic to them.

ANESTHESIA RECOVERY

The cuff of the endotracheal tube should be deflated immediately after the gas is turned off. The tube can be removed as soon as the animal begins to swallow, but a few minutes observation postextubation is warranted, especially if the animal is struggling or distressed. It is best to have a recovery area where animals are in plain sight (e.g., cages in the work area) so that problems can be noted and attended to immediately (Fig. 6-11).

The catheter may be pulled when the animal has recovered to the point where it can control its body in a head-up, sternal position. Opioid antagonists will take effect fastest if they are administered IV while the catheter is still in place.

Heated cages are ideal in the anesthesia recovery area. It should be routine to take the temperatures of postanesthesia animals and to provide heat support

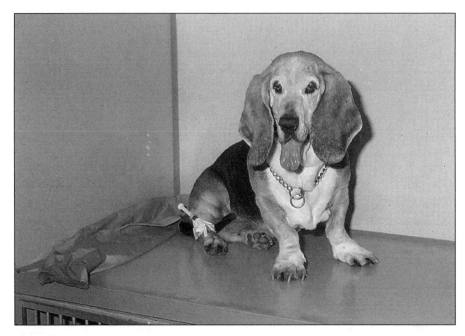

Figure 6-11
Anesthetized animals should recover in heated cages placed where they can be readily observed.

if they are hypothermic. Heat lamps and waterblankets can be brought to the cage of a recovering animal to speed its return to normal body temperature.

The administration of fluids may cause a full bladder, and for the comfort of the animal there should be accommodation for urination as soon as possible after anesthesia. Oftentimes an animal will fuss, and we mistakenly think it is in pain, when the only problem is the need to urinate.

> The careful and safe administration of anesthesia, and diligent attention to the comfort and pain control of the animal after dental procedures, will ensure fast, complete recovery of your patient. Owners will be impressed by the use of analgesic drugs and never complain about paying for them.

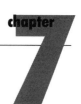

Dental Charting

Perhaps the most important part of a dental prophy is to "chart" an animal's mouth—that is, to create a document that identifies what pathologies exist in the mouth before treatment and what treatment is performed on the animal. In most practices, the technician performs prophies and charts patients unassisted. The charting is a tremendous responsibility because it becomes part of the animal's permanent record and, as such, is a legal document.

Clients are often dissatisfied with dental care, especially if it involves extractions. Most of the dissatisfaction exists because of a lack of communication with the client. An owner presents a pet for a "dental" (A dental what? A dental cleaning? A dental extraction?) and receives an animal several teeth lighter. Regardless of whether you know that the extractions were the best thing for the pet to end pain and infection, the owner sees unauthorized extractions as an invasion of the animal's body (and the owner's pocket). Even if the owner was apprised of the possibility of extractions, he or she could have second thoughts and question their necessity. If the practice cannot provide records to support why the extractions were done (deep periodontal pockets, no gingival attachment, etc.), there is a strong potential for a lawsuit or a malpractice complaint.

Dental charting begins with a form that will allow the technician to record the oral environment of a particular animal at a given time in a complete but shorthand fashion. This is done through abbreviations, written explanations, and marks that visually represent pathologies or therapies. A good dental chart therefore has an accurate depiction of normal teeth so abnormalities can be drawn on it, and it has a large enough format that abbreviations and notes can be made easily. Also, since most dental charts will be used for prophies, they can include a check-off system for charges.

Many practices in the past have tried to severely limit the size of charts to save on storage space. Either they have no record at all, have made a quick note ("dental, extracted three teeth"), or have used a stick-on chart with only the open-mouth (occlusal) view of the teeth.

A full-page chart is necessary for every dental visit. Also, it is critical that there be at least one if not two or more views of the teeth beyond the occlusal. The more important of these additional views is the buccal/labial (the outsides of the teeth) with roots and (my personal bias) an indication of the line of attached gingiva. The second (and less important because there are seldom lesions that must be drawn here) is a view of the insides of the crowns from the lingual/palatal aspect.

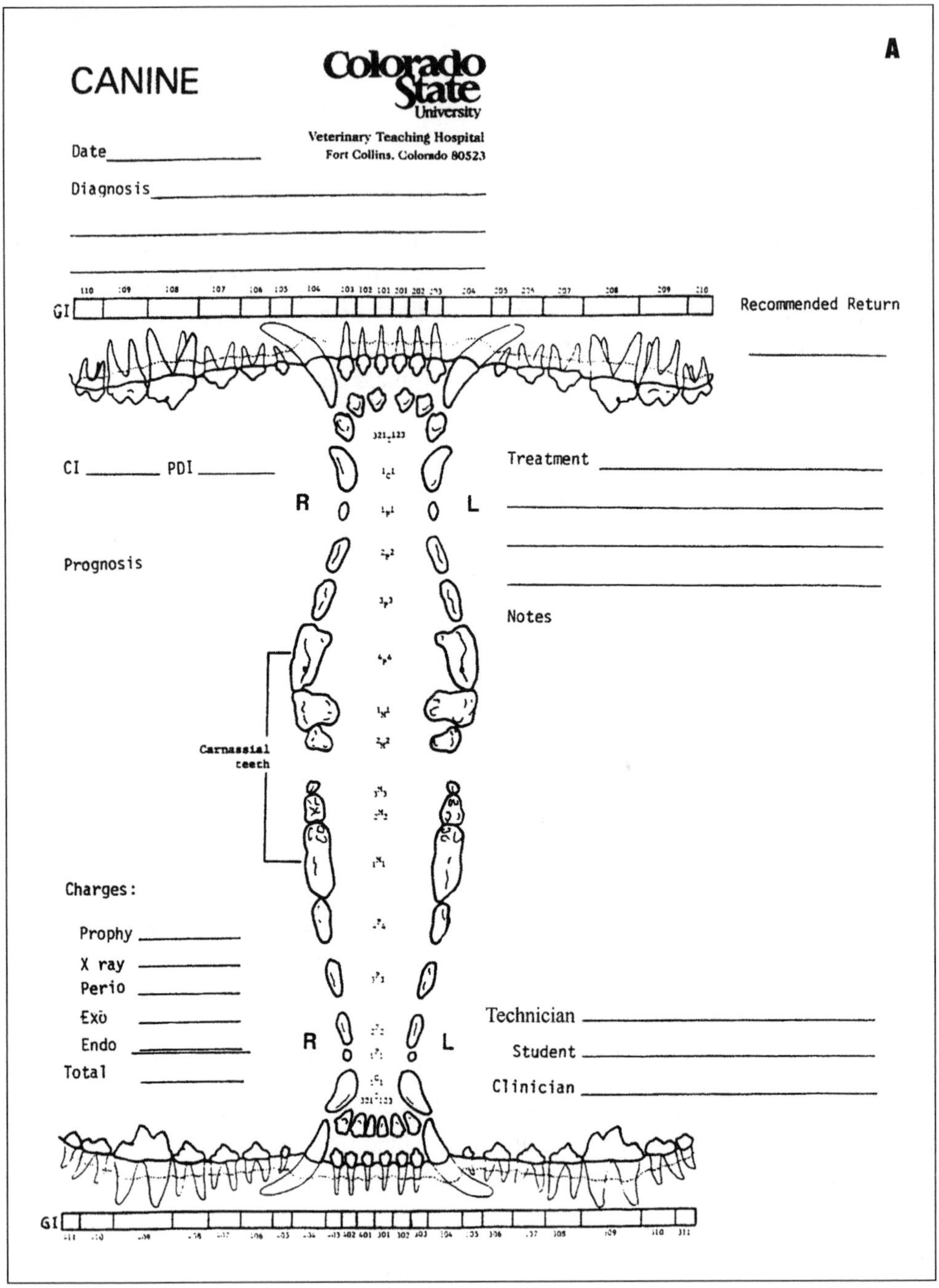

Figure 7-1

The charts developed at CSU for the dog (A) and cat (B). The open-mouth occlusal view is easier to understand for students unfamiliar with the teeth. The teeth are identified by both anatomical and Modified Triadan terminology, and the mucogingival line (MGL) is indicated so that degree of gingival loss or hyperplasia can be drawn in.

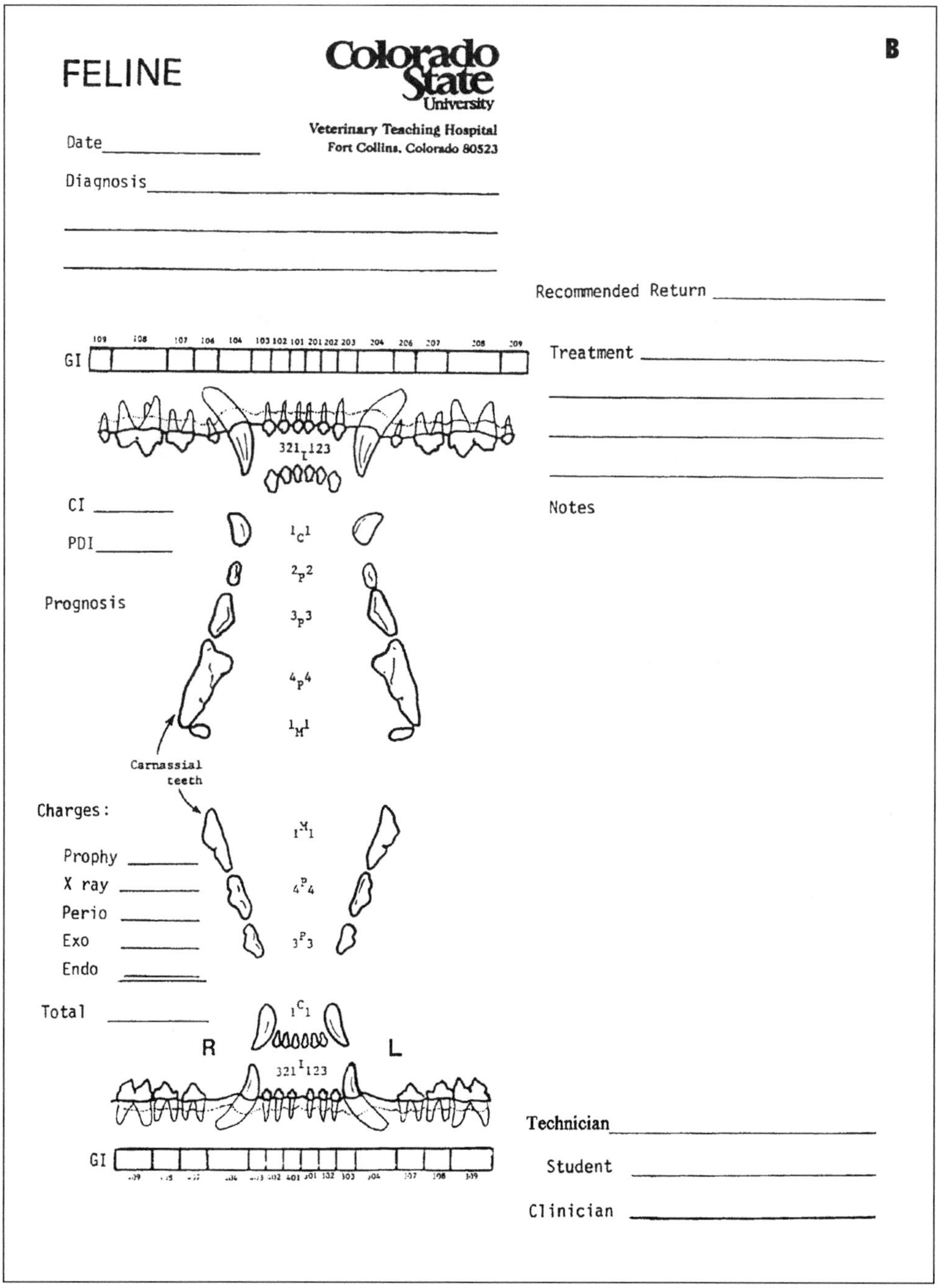

FELINE

Colorado State University
Veterinary Teaching Hospital
Fort Collins, Colorado 80523

Date_____

Diagnosis_____
_____
_____

Recommended Return _____

GI

CI _____
PDI_____

Prognosis

Charges:

Prophy _____
X ray _____
Perio _____
Exo _____
Endo _____

Total _____

Treatment _____
_____
_____
_____

Notes

Carnassial teeth

Technician_____
Student _____
Clinician _____

Figure 7-1 (continued)

123

EDWARD R. EISNER, D.V.M.

Diplomate, Amer. Vet. Dental College
Campus Veterinary Clinic, P.C.
2186 South Colorado Boulevard, Suite C
Denver, Colorado 80222
Phone (303) 757-8481 FAX (303) 759-4729

DENVER VETERINARY DENTAL SERVICE

FELINE

Page _____

Owner & NO. _____
Name _____ Breed _____
Birth Date _____ Sex _____ Color _____
Referred by: _____

Date: _____

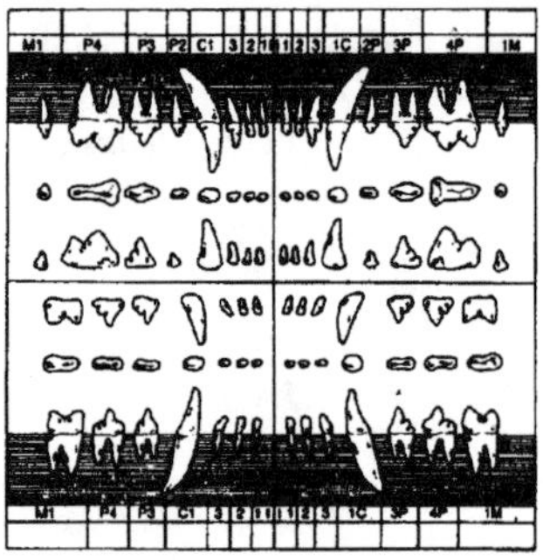

Reason for Visit _____ Diet: _____
Previous Dental History _____
Home Dental Care: Brushing _____ Oral Rinse _____ Medication _____
Other Pertinent History _____
NPO _____ HRS.

EXAMINATION (Gen. Cond. _____; Weight _____ lbs; Heart _____ Color _____ CRT _____)
☐ No Teeth Missing

TREATMENT: VT _____ DVM _____

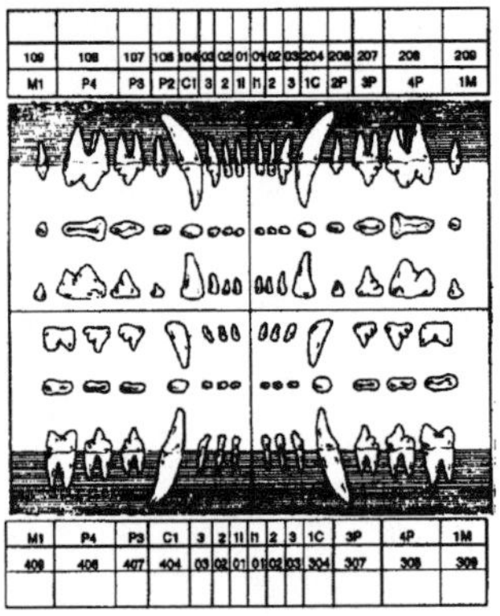

KEY: 0 = Normal   1 = Mild   2 = Moderate   3 = Advanced

Occlusal Evaluation:

Oral Examination (Saliva, Breath, Tonsils, Lnn):

Periodontal Evaluation:

Gingival Index: 0 = Normal, No Swelling.   1 = No Bleeding When Probed
(GI)   2 = Bleeds When Probed   3 = Spontaneous Bleeding

Calculus Index: 0 = No Plaque   1 = Soft Film at Margin
(CI)   2 = Calculus Easily Seen   3 = Heavy Deposits

Endodontic Evaluation:

Radiographic Evaluation:

TREATMENT PLAN:

LIAISON WITH REFERRING DOCTOR
Person contacted   Phone   Record   Person

TREATMENT KEY

ANESTHESIA	TIME	DOSE	AGENT
Preanesthetic			
Anesth. Induct.			
E. T. size		GAS	
End of Procedure			
Support			

PROPHYLAXIS Home Care Instructions _____

1. Ultrasonic cleaning _____   2. Subgingival curettage _____
3. Polishing _____   4. Other _____

ASSESSMENT/ADDITIONAL THERAPY:

Figure 7-2

The canine chart of the Campus Veterinary Clinic, Denver, Colorado. This chart is set up for one side to be used for diagnosis and the other for treatment. *Modified from Steve Holmstrom et al.*, Veterinary Dental Techniques (*Saunders, 1993*).

The dental charts for dogs and cats that were developed for the Veterinary Teaching Hospital at Colorado State University are shown in Figure 7-l. Note that there is no lingual/palatal view. This was purposefully omitted to allow the other views to be as large as possible.

Another popular basic chart, which was developed by Dr. Steve Holmstrom, is presented in Figure 7-2. The most noticeable difference between the two types is the difference in the occlusal view. In the commercial chart the teeth are spread out in a horizontal line, whereas in the CSU chart they are in approximate anatomical position. The anatomical configuration requires more paper space but allows less experienced personnel (notably, veterinary and technical students) to orient themselves more readily to which teeth they are dealing with.

Charting may be done by the person performing the examination during the prophy, or it can be dictated. The advantages of dictation are that the animal need not be kept anesthetized for the extra time that it takes to mark the chart, that gloves do not have to be taken off or hands cleaned in order to keep the chart clean and dry, and that the chart is marked during the prophy and not after because confusion or forgetfulness will lead to errors.

The disadvantages are that another person must be involved (if fleetingly) and that both must have a complete understanding of anatomical or numerical terminology (or preferably, both) and directional terminology. For instance, the clerk should be able to document either of the following lesions in about two seconds each: "a 3 mm gingival recession of the distal buccal root of 208" or "an 8 mm pocket with complete attachment loss of mesial interproximal 304." Yet if these were spelled out on the record, they each would take a great deal more than two seconds, and in a periodontal patient there can easily be as many lesions like this as there are teeth (and sometimes more!).

Note that the numerical system of nomenclature was used here. It is much more efficient to say 403 than "lower right third incisor"—it is less than half as many syllables! However, this only works if both the clerk and the speaker know what is meant, regardless of whether numerical or anatomical terminology is used. It is possible to dictate to an untutored clerk, but the difficulty in telling him or her what to write or draw virtually eliminates the advantage of dictation.

STEPS IN CHARTING: THE DIAGNOSIS

Charting is generally performed one side at a time after teeth are cleaned. Many times it is advantageous to also extract teeth before turning the animal so that repeated turnings are not necessary (the extractions would also be noted, of course—after they are performed).

1. Calculus index. The first step in charting is assignment of a calculus index (CI). A calculus index of 1 means that calculus covers less than one-half of the crown of any tooth. CI2 means the calculus covers more than half of the crown, but not all. In CI3, virtually all of the tooth crown is covered, and calculus is profuse and thickened and extends under the gingiva. These categories are meant to give an impression of the entire mouth. If a single tooth is affected more than the others, such as an upper fourth premolar that has suffered an open slab fracture, causing the dog to avoid chewing on the sensitive tooth, that may be the only tooth with a dentinal surface that is rough with excessive calculus. A notation should be made of the condition of that particular tooth as opposed to the rest of the mouth.

2. Missing teeth. Next is documentation of missing teeth, which are circled on the chart. It makes it less confusing if teeth in both the occlusal and buccal/labial views are circled, although some may prefer to circle only the occlusal view. Noting missing teeth not only establishes that all teeth were examined but could provide important information for the owner.

For instance, if all four second premolars are missing in a Terveren, this is important information for an owner who naively plans to show and breed show-quality puppies from the dog: Lack of a full mouth disqualifies this breed in the show ring, and the trait is heritable. Premolars are the teeth most often missing because of a developmental disorder, so it is critical that the observer be able to count to four (the number of premolars in each quadrant of the mouth of a dog). The simplest way to orient oneself in the rear of the mouth is to look at the carnassial teeth, which are the largest teeth in either jaw. The upper carnassial tooth is the fourth premolar (tooth 108 or 208), and the lower carnassial is the first molar (tooth 309 or 409). You simply count premolars in descending order from these teeth. If there is a tooth missing, there is usually a larger gap, or interproximal space, where it should have been. However, the gap may be very subtle, and sometimes determining which tooth is lacking may depend on radiographs (e.g., is it one- or two-rooted?) or may be an arbitrary choice.

Documenting that a tooth was missing when the dog came in (and letting the owner know) could avoid difficulty in the future if

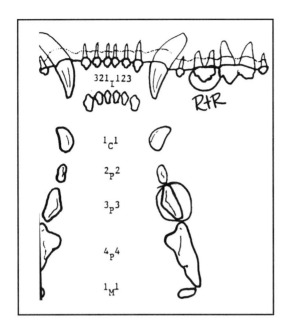

Figure 7-3
The missing tooth is circled on
this cat chart. RtR indicates
there are retained roots.

someone else finds the tooth gone and reports it. The easiest way
to inform the owner is with a modified dental chart with missing
teeth circled.

Roots without a tooth crown are signified by circling only the
crown in the labial/buccal view and writing RtR (for retained root)
next to the tooth (Fig. 7-3). The presence of a root or roots is ver-
ifiable by radiograph. Visible and palpatable evidence is a root
exposed in the gingiva that may be felt only as a "click" when an
instrument or the fingernail is passed over a slightly reddened area.
In a mature animal, retained roots are suspected when there is a
bump under the gingiva where a tooth should be. It also could
mean an erupting tooth in an immature animal, or even an
impacted tooth or a tumor in an older animal. Radiology could
confirm any one of these.

Retained roots occur frequently in cats that have suffered resorptive
lesions with enough tooth destroyed at the neck for the crown to
crack off. The most frequently affected teeth are the third premolars.
Retained roots can also result from trauma or improper or incomplete
extractions, and if these cause pathology later on (abscesses or
gingival inflammation), whoever did the extraction is accountable.

However, there is no way to determine whether a feline retained root was due to a resorptive lesion or an extraction that went awry, which is unfortunately an argument for not documenting your cases if sloppy extractions are performed!

Extractions are documented only after they are performed, and it is critical to indicate the correct tooth (see below).

3. Malformed and malpositioned teeth. Any malformed or malpositioned teeth should be documented. The best way is to draw the tooth as it presents itself, but if you are unable to do this, a notation would be appropriate. A tooth in which the crown appears to have attempted to double itself but is still fused at the base or neck of the tooth is termed "dilacerated" (DL). However, many other malformations occur that may require descriptive language or artistic talent, or both. More common malpositions of teeth may be shown on the chart several ways. One is as a drawn-over outline in a contrasting color of ink. The tooth may also be drawn in the abnormal position after using correction fluid on the chart to obliterate the normal position. If rotation alone has occurred, a curved arrow showing approximate rotation can be drawn.

4. Supernumerary teeth. Extra teeth should be drawn into the chart in their approximate position (Fig. 7-4). It may be necessary to consult with the veterinarian or another knowledgeable person if you are unsure which tooth is duplicated because there are times when it is very difficult to tell which is the extra tooth. In some cases the extra tooth is a deciduous ("baby") tooth. A deciduous tooth will always look different on an X ray, so radiology may be required, particularly before extracting it.

5. Traumatized teeth. Fractured teeth should be noted on the chart. A fracture that extends only through enamel or dentin is a closed fracture (FxC); one that extends into the pulp is an open fracture (FxO). For open fractures it should be indicated whether the pulp is alive or dead, that is, vital (V) or nonvital (NV). For the most part the open fractures seen will be nonvital, and the exposed pulp chamber will be dark or black and will not bleed when entered with the dental explorer. The dog or cat will not flinch when the dental explorer enters a dead tooth either, unless the tooth is abscessing at the root apex, causing pain every time the tooth is

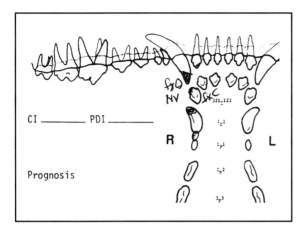

CI _____ PDI _____

Prognosis

Figure 7-4

This dog was found to have a supernumerary (extra) first premolar and both a closed (FxC) and open (FxO) fracture. The addition of V for vital or NV for nonvital for open fractures completes the diagnosis.

touched. Indicating the shape of the lost section of crown will make a more meaningful pictorial record. The missing crown can be blacked out, or crosshatching can be utilized to show the extent of a slab fracture on the side view of a tooth. The location of a pulp exposure can be drawn in.

Other traumatized teeth may be discolored without loss of crown structure. These can simply be noted by number in a narration on the side or indicated by an arrow. The color is important for the prognosis of the tooth. A pink or lilac color may indicate a live tooth that will fade in time; a gray coloration may indicate a dead tooth. You should be as descriptive as possible with the color.

6. Gingival index. Describing the periodontal health of the patient is a critical notation. First is the gingival index (GI). If the gingiva has flat, tapered margins and is a healthy pink (except where the gingiva is pigmented, which is normal in some breeds), the gingival index is 0, or no mark. If the margins are at all swollen or rounded, or if there is reddening at the margins, the index is 1. If there is enough inflammation that the gingiva bleeds when the periodontal probe is passed gently along the deepest part of the sulcus, the index is a 2. If there is gingival hyperplasia, ulceration, signs of severe inflammation (as might occur in stomatitis in cats), or spontaneous bleeding, the index is 3. A gingival index may be given for the entire mouth or for individual teeth.

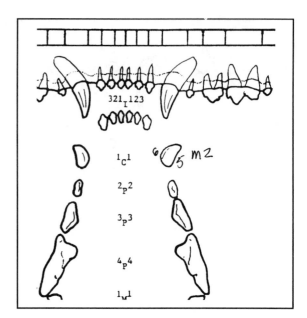

Figure 7-5

Movement in a tooth is indicated by M1, M2, or M3, depending on how much the tooth moves.

7. Stomatitis and kissing ulcers. The inflammation of stomatitis should be described and drawn on the chart as much as possible. Otherwise there will be no way of telling how the lesions are progressing or receding over time, especially if the same person cannot examine the animal. One way is to outline the extent of the lesions, and another is to shade in with light crosshatching. The presence of a "kissing ulcer" or other oral mucosal ulceration should be noted and located on the chart. Kissing ulcers are erosive lesions in tissues where they touch severe periodontal lesions or calculus, as in the area of the cheek that lays over a severely infected upper first molar.

8. Tooth mobility. Mobility of teeth usually results from periodontitis but can be a result of other conditions, such as a recent trauma, fractured root, orthodontic movement, lack of adequate alveolar bone (as in lower incisors), and so on. Dental sulcus measurements and the presence of infection will determine if the problem is periodontal. Movement is graded 1, 2, or 3 (Fig. 7-5). M1 is barely detectable movement, generally less than 1 mm at the tip of the crown when the tooth is pushed; M2 is obvious movement in a tooth that appears to be held fast in the alveolus; and M3 is a floppy tooth that can in some cases be accidently extracted when it is

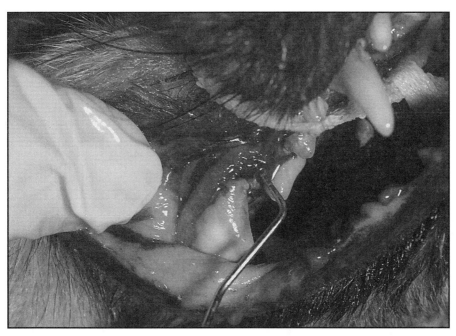

Figure 7-6
The periodontal probe is gently "walked" along the inside of the gingival sulcus to palpate for pockets. Depths that exceed about 4 mm in a large dog, 2 mm in a small dog, and 1 mm in a cat are pathological and should be noted. A narrow-tipped probe should be used on small dogs and cats.

pushed. No movement is M0, but as for most conditions, the normal is simply left blank.

9. Probing depth. The gingival sulcus is the space formed between the tooth and the free gingival margin. Its depth around each tooth needs to be measured with the periodontal probe (Fig. 7-6) as one means of determining the periodontal index (PDI). In general, dogs have a normal gingival sulcus of 4 mm or less, and cats have a normal sulcus of a millimeter or less. Very small dogs, less than 10 lb, should have sulci of 2 mm or less. One way to tell what a normal sulcular depth should be is to check the sulcus of the lower first molar. Many times this is the healthiest gingiva in the mouth because of the tooth constantly being cleaned by the scissors action with the upper carnassial. However, this is not always true. This tooth can be very seriously affected, to the point of pathological jaw fracture from severe periodontal infection of the roots.

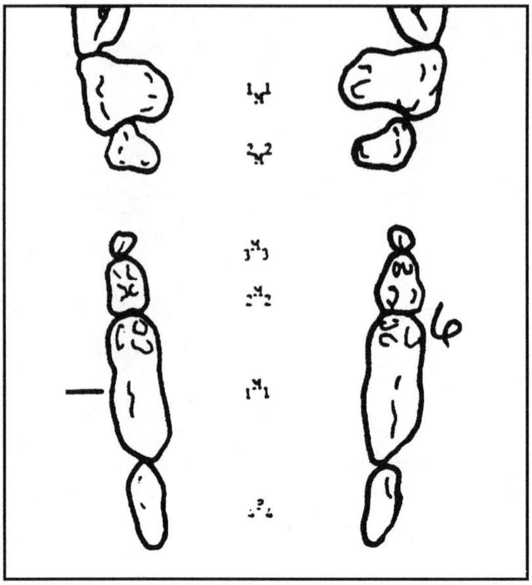

Figure 7-7

A 6-mm pocket that would not be evident without probing is indicated on the occlusal view. If the pocket can be cleaned to its full extent, and there is still attached gingiva, the tooth may be saved. Without treatment of the subgingival root area, the periodontal attachments will eventually be lost.

The periodontal probe should be placed gently to the bottom of the sulcus, which becomes a periodontal pocket (by definition) if the depth exceeds normal (Fig. 7-7). The normal depth is just to the CEJ (cemento-enamel junction), the area where the crown meets the root. When periodontal infection erodes the tissues at the CEJ, the probing depth increases. The probe should be "walked" around the tooth to measure at least four spots for a single-rooted tooth (mesial, distal, labial, and lingual or palatal). For a multirooted tooth at least one additional measurement should be taken over each additional root. Only the abnormal measurements should be noted, so for a healthy mouth there will be no periodontal pocket numbers at all. The numbers for pocket depth are written next to the tooth on the occlusal (open mouth) view in the position they were measured.

Often the periodontal probe will reveal probing depths that were not noticed when a tooth was scaled, and these may require further deep root cleaning (root planing) if the tooth is not extracted. Closed root planing (RPC) should be noted at this time so that it is not forgotten. Take heed that a periodontal pocket deeper than 6 mm is considered too deep to adequately clean without cutting and flapping the gingiva for visualization of the root (which is open root planing, or RPO). If the notation RPC was used to identify an 8-mm pocket, the work would be suspect.

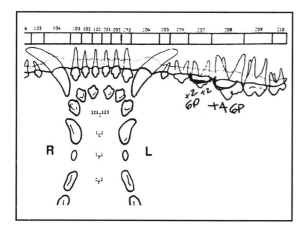

Figure 7-8
Excessive growth of gingiva due to inflammation (gingival hyperplasia) is indicated on the labial/buccal views of the teeth. The estimated length beyond normal is indicated (as in +4), and the approximate shape drawn on the chart. The excessive tissue must be amputated to normal length with a tapering cut; restoring the length of free gingiva is called gingivoplasty, indicated on the chart by GP.

10. Gingival recession and hyperplasia. A second measurement should be made for any gingival recession or gingival hyperplasia on the labial/buccal view of the teeth. The periodontal probe is used to measure as before, but it is not inserted into the sulcus or pocket. The free gingival margin should lap over the tooth crown about 2 mm in most portions of dogs' mouths. If the actual margin has receded, an estimate is made for how far it has receded. For instance, if there are 3 mm of root exposed, there are about 5 mm of recession. However, for teeth that have normally deeper sulcus depths (like the upper canine), 3 mm of exposed root may represent 7 mm of recession. Sometimes the gingiva on the tooth on the other side of the mouth is normal by comparison, and sometimes there is an obvious divot in the line of the gingival margin so that it is easy to imagine and measure to where the margin should be.

A line should be drawn in the approximate area of the receded margin over the affected root, and next to that a number written to represent the amount of recession. An advantage of having the mucogingival line already on the chart is that drawing the line of recession beyond this automatically indicates that attached gingiva is completely lost. Complete attachment loss should be noted explicitly, however, because it is grounds for extractions. The abbreviation for attachment loss is AL.

Gingival hyperplasia, or hypertrophy, is the opposite situation (Fig. 7-8). Here the margin has increased in length over the tooth. To estimate how much longer it is than normal, the normal shape should be gauged. For this, the existing approximate shape relative to the size of the teeth is drawn, and a notation of additional length is made next to it (e.g., +4, for plus 4 mm). Note that large hypertrophic masses must be amputated to allow adequate cleaning of the crown and subgingival area; these are gingivoplasties (GVPs). If a hypertrophic mass extends 8 mm over the tooth beyond the normal gingival margin without any attachment loss at the CEJ (which is rare, but not unknown), a pseudopocket exists. Usually pseudopockets and true periodontal pockets appear in the same mouth, sometimes over the same tooth. Obviously, with a combination of pocket depths on the occlusal portion of the chart and hyperplasia on the labial/buccal, you can indicate the true depth that you probed, e.g., 6 (occlusal) and +7 (labial) amounts to 13 mm.

11. Furcation. A condition commonly seen with gingival recession is the result of the periodontal loss of alveolar bone in the space between roots. This space is called the furcation, and the periodontal lesions in this area are called furcation lesions. They are graded 1, 2, or 3. The F1 is a depression in the furcation area that extends less than halfway under the crown. If the depression extends more than halfway through, but not all the way, it is an F2. When the gingiva and bone are missing completely and the periodontal probe can be passed from one side to the other, it is an F3.

12. Periodontal index. The assessment of the condition of the gingiva, the presence or absence of stomatitis or oral ulceration, the probing depths, and measurements of the gingiva and associated degree of infection in the periodontal tissues allows a qualitative assessment of periodontitis, called the periodontal index (PDI). The periodontal index is measured from 1 to 4. It is somewhat subjective but can be summarized as follows.

A PDI1 is essentially gingivitis alone, without attachment loss. The gingiva, of course, is the first tissue to show the effects of infection and inflammation.

As periodontitis progresses, the attachment at the CEJ is lost, and infection begins to progress along the tooth roots toward the root apices. PDI2 indicates less than 25 percent attachment loss. This is a general assessment of the condition of the mouth. If only one or two teeth have periodontitis more severe, it should probably be made plain that this condition is localized to teeth x and y. In PDI2, gingiva is definitely inflamed, and minimal recession has occurred, or very shallow pockets (13 mm) have formed. The condition is most obvious in the most susceptible areas, such as between the upper fourth premolar and the first molar or between the lower first and second molars. On radiographs, bone loss is slight or negligible. Oral malodor (halitosis) is present but is usually merely unpleasant, not overwhelming.

When the periodontal index has progressed to the third level (PDI3), the lesions are more advanced and more generalized in the mouth. Attachment loss is 25–50 percent. Pockets and recessions are not only slightly deeper but the gingiva often shows some hyperplasia or reveals the beginnings of free pus. Radiographs show significant horizontal and vertical bone loss, and oral malodor is distinctly redolent of death and rotting.

PDI3 represents the imminent loss of teeth. Here is where the complete loss of gingival attachment is seen on some teeth and where extractions or periodontal surgeries are first required. Some teeth are mobile because of periodontal destruction, including teeth with more than one root. Oral odor is objectionable, and there is free pus present around some tooth roots.

PDI4 represents very serious periodontitis, with greater than 50 percent attachment loss and teeth that may exfoliate (fall out). Carnassials or canine teeth, despite their considerable length and size of roots, may have enough attachment loss to show mobility. Oronasal fistulas on the medial aspect of the upper canines are common in some breeds due to periodontal infection. Radiographs show both horizontal and vertical bone loss. Combination periodontal/endodontal abscessation may be present because of complete loss of attachment to the apices of roots. Ulceration and purulent exudation of gingiva and mucosa are common, and pus flows from around roots. Sometimes the skin at the commissures of the lips or areas where the animal licks is afflicted with dermatitis from oral bacteria. Osteomyelitis (infection of the bone) may have resulted in tumorous-appearing bony swelling of the face or jaw. Spontaneous mandibular fractures due to lysis of bone around tooth roots (particularly around the rostral root of the lower first molar) occur. The gingiva and mucosa are typically brick red and exudative. The attitude of the animal is usually noticeably affected by the infection in the mouth, and there may be problems in other organs due to spreading of the infection. Blood work usually indicates a chronic disease condition. The animal either refuses food entirely, bolts it without chewing, or will only eat soft food. The oral odor is almost overwhelming. Periodontal abscessation may result in facial or mandibular soft tissue swelling.

It is worth saying to clients that PDI1 corresponds with gingivitis (mild, moderate, or severe) and PDI2, 3, and 4 correspond with mild, moderate, and severe periodontitis.

13. Other findings. If radiographs are used for diagnostics, they should be noted on the chart. Radiographic findings should be written out as comments. For instance, if full-survey X rays were taken and found to be normal, the note "X rays, survey, normal" would quickly impart the information. If a problem was suspected in an upper canine, you could write "X ray, rostral maxilla, 104, increased pulp chamber with apical lucency." This would indicate a dead tooth that had been nonvital for some time (because the opposite canine's pulp chamber had continued to narrow but the affected tooth's had not) with an apical abscess. Any other comments that would help make the chart clear should be included so that when the dental chart is read at a later date a mental picture of the mouth can easily be constructed.

CHARTING DENTAL THERAPIES

Although recording therapy beyond a dental prophy is properly the responsibility of the veterinarian who performs it, there may be situations where the veterinarian prefers to have the technician act as clerk and recorder. Some charts are all-inclusive; the diagnosis and therapy are shown on the same form. Some have two forms so that diagnoses or findings can fit on one and therapies on the other. Each has advantages and disadvantages, and each practice must choose which is the most convenient to use.

1. Extractions. Extractions are obviously the most frequent therapy for dental patients. All extractions must be signified by an × over the tooth in the occlusal view (Fig. 7-9). Duplicating the × on the tooth on the labial/buccal view makes the chart more complete.

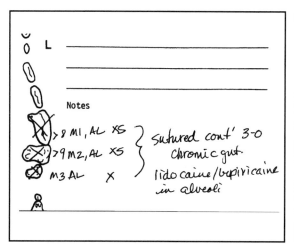

Notes

> 8 M1, AL ✗S
> 9 M2, AL ✗S
M3 AL   ✗

} sutured cont' 3-0
chronic gut.
lidocaine/bupivicaine
in alveoli

Figure 7-9

Extractions of teeth are indicated by an x through each tooth. Next to the tooth should be the reasons for extraction (deep periodontal pockets, complete attachment loss of gingiva [AL], endodontal abscess due to open fracture, etc.). Also next to the tooth should be an indication of simple extraction (x), sectioned extraction (xs), or surgical extraction (xss). For legal reasons, suture type and pattern can be added, and any local or regional blocks specified.

In addition, the types of extractions are noted. There are three: simple, sectioned, and surgical. Simple extractions are single-rooted teeth that are simply elevated and then pulled with forceps (or multirooted teeth that are so loose that they can be pulled without sectioning). Simple extractions are signified by **x**. Cutting the crown to separate it into cusps or sections that correspond to the roots and then elevating each root separately like a simple extraction is represented by **xs**. When gingiva and mucosa need to be elevated and bone cut to extract a tooth, it becomes a surgical extraction, or **xss**. The easiest way to keep track of these is to abbreviate the type of extraction next to the occlusal view of the tooth (or in a box corresponding to the tooth). Since sectioned and surgical extractions involve increasingly more time and effort, they are usually more costly to the client, so keeping track of them is critical to practice income. If gingival sutures are used, this should be noted also (type of suture and pattern).

2. Periodontics. As mentioned above, root planing should be noted on the chart next to the periodontal pocket measurement. The notation RPC (closed root plane) is used when the root surface of the pocket is scraped clean with a curette without the gingiva being surgically removed (Fig. 7-10). If the veterinarian raises a gingival flap for open root planing, it becomes RPO. If she or he must recontour bone to make a smooth base for the reattached gingiva, it is an alveoloplasty, or AP.

Figure 7-10

Any pocket that is in excess of the normal 4 mm in a dog should have the exposed root debrided with a curette or ultrasonic scaler. The curette is the only tool with which you can feel the roughness of subgingival calculus or an eroded root surface. All calculus and necrotic debris must be cleaned out if the gingiva is to be allowed to reattach. This therapy is root planing (RP). If the pocket is 6 mm or less, it may be done with the gingiva in place and is called closed root planing (RPC); if the gingiva must be incised and elevated in a flap to get to the depths of the pocket, it is called open root planing (RPO).

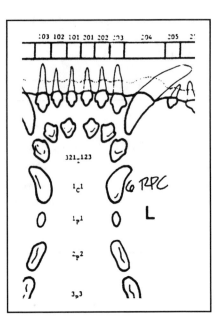

A gingivoplasty should be indicated by GVP next to the drawing of the hypertrophied tissue.

There are numerous other abbreviations for periodontal therapies, but these are probably used so seldom that they are just as easy to spell out as to look up each time. A list of abbreviations approved by the American Veterinary Dental College may be found in Appendix 3.

If a therapeutic product is used on periodontal tissues, it should be noted (e.g., Heska perioceutic).

3. Endodontics. A root canal may be conventional (RC) or surgical (RCS), in which mucosa is excised and the apex of the root is exposed for amputation (apicoectomy) and seal. Another endodontal therapy that is frequently performed is pulp capping (PC), also known as a vital pulpotomy. Cutting crowns to prevent them from traumatizing other structures or for disarming purposes is a crown amputation (CAM). Crown amputation is almost always coupled with a pulp cap

(CAM/PC) since removal of more than a couple of millimeters of crown will cause pulp exposure.

Endodontic procedures often require a narrative. For instance, for a pulp cap, the thickness of calcium hydroxide powder, intermediate restoration material, and final restoration should be noted, as well as what type of restoration materials are used. This will allow the veterinarian to assess the long-term efficacy of techniques and materials.

4. Other. One abbreviation for a therapy that may be seen often is OP, odontoplasty. This technique is frequently used to smooth the edges or surfaces of the crown when a fracture has occurred. It has both aesthetic and practical functions because a rough crown will collect calculus and will induce gingival inflammation if it is not smooth under the free gingiva. A sharp edge may also cause abrasions to the lip, cheek, or tongue. Any restorations or crown treatments should be noted.

The overall reason for charting is to remember exactly what was seen and what was done at a visit. It is meant to allow personnel in the practice to see trends in dental care and the results of the care. It is also a legal document that will support proper dental diagnosis and therapy.

Assisting with Extractions

Depending on the skill of the technician and the practice law of a particular state, the veterinarian may call on the technician to perform certain extractions or may ban technician extractions entirely. In many states the practice act is quite specific, and tooth extraction is considered a surgical technique; as such, it is limited to veterinarians licensed in the state. In other locales, the practice act allows any function of a veterinarian (including surgery) to be performed by another person as long as that person is directly supervised by a veterinarian. Generally this is defined as the veterinarian being on the premises rather than necessarily physically watching the procedure. The veterinarian is responsible for any procedure done under his or her license, so few are going to authorize a technician to do complicated surgical extractions. The description of more complicated extractions (sectioned and surgical) are included here to aid the technician in preparing for and assisting in these procedures.

There are several indications for extraction of teeth. The most frequent indication is teeth that have serious periodontal compromise (Fig. 8-1). Extraction would also be the choice of treatment for a tooth that was fractured longitudinally (along its length) from the mouth into the root so that a seal of the pulp was impossible. When a fractured tooth could be treated endodontically, an owner may elect to extract it because of cost or because of the animal's habits (it keeps chewing things that break teeth).

Other indications include fractures that involve bone, in which the blood supply to the bone has been compromised. Such bone becomes (with the tooth) a sequestrum, which is an island of dead tissue surrounded by live tissue. Tiny pieces of bone may lose their vitality, and the surrounding bone tissue will mobilize to clean up the dead tissue and replace it with new bone. However, when the piece is large enough, it is prone to contamina-

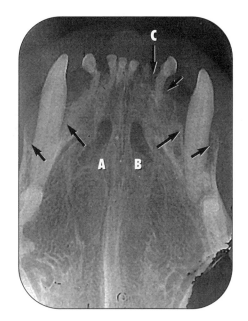

Figure 8-1

Serious periodontal lesions can be confirmed by X ray. Widening of the periodontal ligament space indicates deep involvement of the periodontal ligament, as in these upper canines in a cat (A and B). Also note the loss of bone around the third incisor (C).

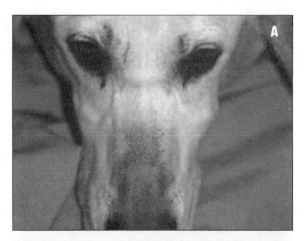

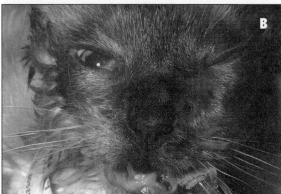

Figure 8-2

Endodontal abscesses (A and B) may occur due to even small fractures into the pulp chamber through the crown, and if owners do not elect root canal therapy, the teeth should be extracted. Periodontal disease (C) may progress to the tooth root to destroy the blood and nerve supply to the tooth pulp and cause a similar-looking abscess (arrow); such a tooth must always be extracted since there is no way to seal off infection.

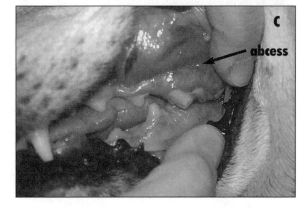

tion with bacteria, either from the outside world or from those that may be circulating in the blood, which sets up a chronic, nonhealing draining abscess.

Additional indications for extraction include supernumerary (extra) or malpositioned teeth, teeth crowded from the mouth being too small, or retained deciduous teeth. Abscessation from endodontal disease (Fig. 8-2) can be so severe that

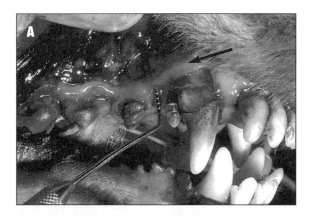

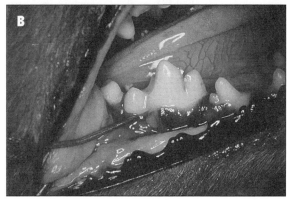

Figure 8-3

(A) Palpation of deep periodontal pockets in two
dogs.

(B) The complete loss of
attachment shown here
lends a grim prognosis
for a tooth.

roots are resorbed; these teeth are not candidates for root canal therapy and so should be extracted. In cats, teeth with stage 2 and 3 resorptive lesions should be extracted because they are painful and the affected teeth are doomed.

The multitude of reasons for extractions also suggests that there are both very easy and very difficult extractions. A tooth that has been chronically abscessing may have a soft apical abscess but extensive ankylosis (bone crossing the periodontal ligament because of inflammation and then bonding to the tooth root) along much of the root; such a tooth can be a nightmare to extract. A tooth in which the periodontal attachment has been eaten away by periodontitis and that is only being held in by soft tissues is easy to extract (Fig. 8-3), although the degree of bone loss can lead to pathological fracture (see "Surgical Extractions" below). Very old dogs often have very hard, unyielding bones and brittle teeth that are difficult to extract. Clearly, extraction refers to many types of procedures.

Extraction of teeth needs to be billed on a sliding scale of difficulty. One way to do this is to place extractions into three categories—simple, sectioned, and surgical—and to assess each extraction in a category by how easy or difficult it is.

SIMPLE EXTRACTIONS

The "simple" in simple extractions does not necessarily mean they are easy. Instead it refers to the fact that the target teeth are single rooted and extraction involves only elevating the tooth, not cutting the bone. In the dog the teeth that are subject to simple extractions are the incisors and first premolars. In the cat simple extractions are performed on incisors, upper second premolars and first molars, upper canines, and occasionally, with severe periodontitis, lower canines.

The equipment for simple extractions are few. The first tool needed is an elevator that fits the neck of the tooth (elevators generally come in two sizes, larger for dogs and smaller for cats, very small dogs, or the lower first incisors of larger dogs).

The next instrument needed is a surgical blade (usually the thin, pointed number 11) on a scalpel handle to incise the soft tissue attachment at the cemento-enamel junction (CEJ); however, many people prefer to use the elevator to break down the gingival attachment.

The third instrument that is indicated is an extraction forceps, "pliers" that can grasp the tooth after the elevator has loosened it, although many teeth will come out with the elevator alone. The long-jawed type of extraction forceps used for incisors in humans (there are many styles) are useful for all of the teeth of cats and dogs; the broader, shorter forceps designed for molars in humans are not compatible with animal teeth.

If the attached gingiva is to be raised to slide over the extraction site, a periosteal elevator may be desired (although a sharp dental elevator can do the same job).

Finally, if the extraction site(s) is to be sutured, needle holders, thumb forceps, scissors, and absorbable suture material should be laid out. Infected tissue should be curetted (scraped) out of an extraction site. The soft granulomas that often sit in the alveolus, plus soft, infected bone, must be removed for fast healing. To a certain extent, the elevator (isn't the elevator a useful instrument?) can do this, but excavators to access the alveolus would be convenient.

The following supplies should be on hand as well. If the lip needs to be held back, a retractor should be available. A small Senn retractor works well. One or two surgical towels keep hair out of extraction sites; they are applied to the lips with towel clamps. A quantity of gauze sponges are needed to keep a site blood-free for visualization, and the air/water syringe should be available to rinse the site. A syringe of disinfectant solution and another of local anesthetic completes the setup. The only addition to extraction equipment for sectioned and surgical extractions is a dental drill and all-purpose or cutting burs.

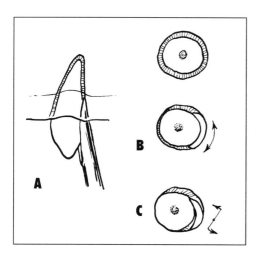

Figure 8-4

There are two ways to apply force in tooth extraction, through the wedge and the lever.

(A) The root elevator acts as a wedge when it is inside the socket, and simply by its presence pushes the tooth out.

(B) Short, rotating motions are used to help the elevator cut through periodontal ligament fibers to advance toward the root apex.

(C) The elevator can also be used as a lever by twisting it within the socket to apply even more force on the periodontal fibers.

The procedure for the extraction is straightforward. If the connection at the CEJ is to be severed, it is done first. If the attached gingiva will be elevated from bone, it should be done before the tooth is extracted because it is more difficult to find the edge of the alveolus when the tooth is gone. As for the actual elevation of the tooth, the elevator is placed tight to the tooth neck as far mesial or distal as possible (see Chap. 1 for definitions of these directions). It is very seldom an option to place the elevator inside the mouth because of the interference of the opposite jaw. This is not necessarily true for the incisors, but with incisors the inside (lingual or palatal) position has the same disadvantage as that of the outside (labial) surface: the leading edge of the bone of the alveolus is so thin that the elevator "skips" over it, to slide under soft tissue alone. We want the elevator to work down the periodontal ligament, and the only place we can do this consistently is squarely on top of the alveolar crest, i.e., mesially or distally.

The elevator mostly acts as a wedge for the extraction (Fig. 8-4A). The tooth root is essentially a cone-shaped structure within a cone-shaped hole (the alveolus). When the elevator is forced down the periodontal ligament space, the natural result is for the root to pop out of the hole, which has become too small for the root when the elevator is wedged inside.

But this is an oversimplification. First, the elevator is pressed into the periodontal ligament space tight to the tooth and pointing to the anticipated tip of the root. If pointed too much toward the tooth, the elevator will come up against hard dentin and make no progress; if pointed more straight down into the bone, it will first gouge through dense cortical and then cancellous bone. Either way the tooth will not move, and in the second case the bone will be damaged unnecessarily.

Once the periodontal ligament is found, there are two motions that can be used. Short, rotating movements will help sever periodontal ligament fibers and allow the elevator to plunge deep into the socket (Fig. 8-4B). A second motion, carefully applied, adds leverage. By keeping the elevator in one place in the socket, but twisting it slightly, even more force can be applied to the periodontal ligament (Fig. 8-4C). The longitudinal levering motion should be applied carefully and held for several seconds. This gives the elastic periodontal ligament fibers the opportunity to stretch and fatigue (lose their strength). If the elevator is used aggressively, especially in older animals, the root will typically break because the pulp is no longer functional and the dentin is brittle.

The combination of the wedge and lever is almost always successful in elevating the single-rooted teeth listed above. Elevating teeth is an activity that requires patience and finesse. It should never be hurried.

Even with careful elevation, occasionally a root tip will fracture off. Usually this can be retrieved with a smaller elevator or a root tip pick placed right at the edge of the root tip and then delicately moved apically. Aggressiveness here in the maxilla may force the root tip into the nasal cavity, into a sinus, or through the cortex; in the lower jaw it could be forced into the mandibular canal. If there is any doubt about the ability to elevate, a surgical retrieval of the root may be called for (see below).

If there is any doubt that a root tip has actually been extracted (and doubts will arise!), an X ray may be used to determine this, or it may help locate where the root tip has been shoved. Then it becomes the decision of the veterinarian as to whether the root tip should be retrieved. If a root is endodontally infected, a root tip will invariably abscess. The act of elevation takes oral and periodontal bacteria up to the root tip even if they weren't there to begin with. Thus contaminated, the root tip tends to become a sequestrum if it is of any size at all. Sometimes long-term antibiotics will save this situation, but for the most part roots must be removed in their entirety; this is a standard of veterinary care. It is generally much easier to do it at the time of the extraction, rather than at a second procedure later on. If a client takes the animal to another hospital for the root tip extraction, he or she may expect the first hospital to pay for the procedure (and may win in court or with a malpractice complaint to the state board of veterinary medicine).

As mentioned above, highly contaminated extraction sites will need to be cleaned of any infected soft tissue and degenerated bone. It is then prudent to lavage with an antimicrobial solution of chlorhexidine, povidone-iodine, or another disinfectant that will be gentle on tissues (see Chap. 5).

Suturing extraction sites that are very small often causes more trauma than the extractions. The extraction site of a small tooth tends to develop a blood

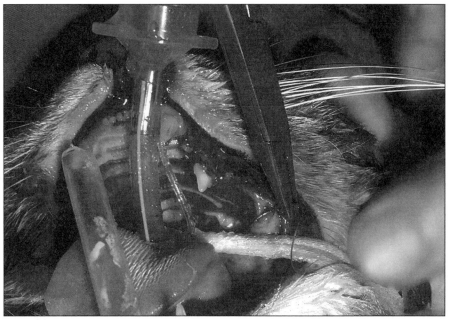

Figure 8-5
Unless they are very small, extraction sites that are sutured heal faster, resulting in more comfort for the animal. Grossly infected material should be removed to normal gingival tissue and normal bleeding bone before suturing.

clot that fills the alveolus until it is replaced with fibrous tissue, which will later be largely replaced by bone. However, if several adjacent incisors are extracted, for instance, there will be a fairly large area of bone exposed. Bone does not fare well if exposed to the saliva of the mouth. Saliva lacks sodium and other solutes in the blood and the intercellular fluid. This hypo-osmolality of saliva, as well as the bacteria in the mouth, leads to the painful condition of alveolar osteitis. In humans, this condition is called dry socket: the protective blood clot is lost from an alveolus after an extraction, which results in painful inflammation of the alveolar bone. Presumably, pets could be suffering from alveolar osteitis more than we imagine. At any rate, unless they are very small, extraction sites that are sutured heal faster (Fig. 8-5).

Suture materials should be absorbable. The best choice, on balance, is chromic gut. Although gut is weaker to tie and handle than synthetic absorbables, there is little holding power in the poorly keratinized gingiva and mucosa that is being sutured, and tension on these tissues will merely pull through anyway. The synthetic absorbables also tend to last too long and sometimes distress the owners by their presence weeks beyond healing after extraction, although they seldom cause a problem for the animals.

In general, tapered needles are preferred to cutting because cutting needles have a tendency to cut through these tissues, gingiva in particular. However, sometimes a cutting needle works better if the gingiva has become very fibrous due to inflammation. Since the tissues tear very easily, and all that is desired is to oppose the edges to allow quicker healing to occur, it is usually best to take a bite on one side, pull the needle through, and then take the bite on the other side. Otherwise, the needle tends to tear through the first side as the tissue is stretched to get to the second. The pattern of sutures (simple interrupted, cruciate, simple continuous) is probably unimportant and is usually a matter of preference of the surgeon. Healing occurs very quickly, and the suture line does not need to remain for a long time. However, it important to make five or six throws (2.5 to 3 square knots), since the wet oral environment tends to allow knots to untie.

SECTIONED EXTRACTIONS

The sectioned extraction is very similar to the simple. The difference is that the target tooth must be cut between the roots to the surface of the bone. The simplest way to visualize the furcation between the roots is to elevate the gingiva before sectioning the tooth, which will reveal the divot in the crown that indicates the beginning of the roots. Almost all teeth with more than one root require sectioning (that is, everything distal to the first premolar in both jaws in the dog, except for the lower third molar, which is almost always single rooted). In the cat, everything caudal to the canine except the second upper premolar and the upper molar will need to be sectioned.

Exceptions to this rule include cases of severe periodontitis, in which teeth are wobbling freely in the alveoli; everyone who has worked on bad mouths has seen this situation, where teeth can be simply flipped out of their alveoli by a flick of the wrist. If there is any doubt, the double- or triple-rooted tooth can be sectioned, or there is likely to be a fractured root tip.

The reason for sectioning is that the roots tend to diverge, rather than simply go straight down, and elevating one root is going to put stress on the other(s) and fracture it(them) (Fig. 8-6). The other important point is that in order to get a two- or three-rooted tooth out intact, the surrounding bone must be collapsed or gouged out, which leads to excessive trauma.

The dental drill is used to section teeth. In a poorly supplied dental operatory, a Dremel-type tool or even a very "low-tech" hacksaw blade (with metal-cutting–sized teeth) can be used here.

In a dental drill the burs used to cut the teeth are tapered fissure-type cutting burs (700 series) or general-purpose pear-shaped burs (330, 331, regular or

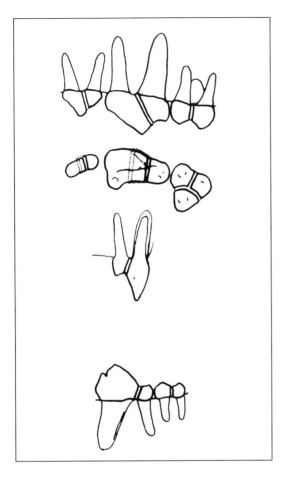

Figure 8-6

Multiple-rooted teeth should be sectioned so that each root may be elevated like a single-rooted tooth, or root fracture will result.

long). The water spray coolant should always be on when the drill is used. Even though the teeth will be discarded and so heat to the tooth need not be a worry (as when the life of the pulp must be retained), the bur causes unwanted heat to the adjacent bone, and the heat generated can reduce the life of burs.

The majority of the cutting surface of all these burs is on the side, so they should always be used in a wiping motion at full speed. The amount of pressure applied should not be enough to unduly slow (or stop) the bur because the high-speed drill cuts most effectively at top speed. Dental drills are high speed but low torque. As air-driven instruments, they rely on the speed rather than mechanical push (torque) to effect the cutting action.

Although there are many situations where a dentist may want a slower drill speed for cutting teeth (which is why drills essentially work in variable speeds according to how much air pressure is released by the foot pedal), for sectioning teeth it should be "pedal to the metal," or full power. Most dental units get the optimum 300,000 rpm with an air supply of between 40 to 60 lb of pressure. If the handpiece is worn or dirty, it takes more pressure to get the drill to speed, and certain brands of handpiece take higher pressures to work efficiently. Experience will tell when the whine of the drill is the right pitch and when it is cutting efficiently.

Once a tooth is sectioned, the elevator is placed between the crown sections and gently twisted. Sometimes this will result in a small "click" as the last little bridge of dentin between the roots snaps. If nothing happens, and the crown seems immobile, the cut is probably not between the roots, or not enough crown has been cut. Usually one portion of the crown moves more than the other; this is the one that should be elevated first.

The roots are individually elevated just like adjacent simple extractions. One should always be exceedingly careful when neighboring teeth that are not to be extracted are contacted by the elevator. Using them to push against can result in their fracture. If there is a need to get between teeth but their crowns are too close for the elevator to fit between, the crown of the doomed tooth is shaved down with   a bur to allow access for the elevator. It may also be necessary to cut bone next to the root with the bur to give a starting purchase for the elevator so that it doesn't slide off the alveolar crest and cut or puncture tissues.

After the roots have been extracted and the alveoli cleaned of necrotic and infected debris, the bone of each alveolus should be assessed for sharpness. The furcation bone in particular, but also other areas of alveolar and surrounding bone, may have projecting sharp edges. The animal will be reluctant to chew if, with every contact in this area, soft tissue is squeezed between food and a sharp bony projection. Eventually this bone will remodel because it is not supported by a tooth. In the meantime the animal can be made more comfortable by cutting off the excess bone with the dental drill, and a more comfortable animal means a more satisfied client. This also may provide some advantage when soft tissue is extended over the extraction site for suturing. Adequate water cooling is definitely necessary for recontouring the bone in an "alveoloplasty" or "osteoplasty" like this because heat will kill the bone, which will result in a necrotic, poorly healing area.

Sometimes, the air from the drill is forced into the bone and creates an air embolus (air bubble in the bloodstream); this has been fatal to a small number of cat and human dental patients (see below).

SURGICAL EXTRACTIONS

Surgical extractions (those that require cutting bone to get roots out) are necessary when lack of access to the root, danger to adjacent structures, tooth root fragility, or ankylosis of the bone to the root exists.

The first situation is commonly found when tooth root tips fracture off. Rather than digging for the root tip blindly, or nearly so, at the bottom of the socket, the root is exposed through the side of the animal's face or mandible by cutting the bone away. Fortunately, except for the roots of the first and second upper incisors, and the medial roots of the first and second molars (which usually are not problems because they are short, blunt roots), all roots are available through the bone of the face or mandible. The gingiva and mucosa are cut and elevated with the periosteum so that the bone covering the tooth root can be incised by the drill with a cutting or all-purpose bur. Once one side of the alveolus is gone, the elevator can be used to simply roll the tooth out.

If it has healthy periodontal attachments, the upper canine of a dog (Fig. 8-7) should never be simply elevated to be extracted because of the high probability of fracturing the thin plate of bone medial to the root (between the root and the nasal passage). This bone, which is typically only about half a millimeter thick, will readily fracture if an elevator is driven medial to the tooth or if, while elevating, the crown of the tooth moves laterally, forcing the root medially into the nose.

The upper canine has a massive root that is longer than the crown. The thin bone of the maxilla over this tooth conforms to the root underneath, and the shape of the root can be appreciated by looking at the swelling (the "juga") of the bone through the thin mucosa. The apex of the root is always at the mesial root of the second premolar, and the tooth is basically banana shaped, being wider in its middle and approximately evenly tapered on either end (the root tip is slightly blunter).

The cortical bone over the tooth is seldom more than a millimeter thick along the entire length of the tooth, which makes outlining the tooth possible without cleaning all of the alveolar and cortical bone off of the surface to see where the root is. The mucosa and gingiva are incised from between the canine and first premolar to the apex of the tooth and along the dental crest to release the soft tissue in a flap. The periosteum will elevate with the gingiva and mucosa, so all soft tissue must be free of the bone before the drill is used.

At the coronal end of the root, the tooth is against palatal bone, which is very dense and tough; this bone must be cut in a trough both mesial and distal to the tooth for about 5 mm along the root (the approximate width of the palatal bone in an average dog). Then the root can simply be outlined by the bur, merely cutting through the cortical plate of bone on the margin of the root (about 2 mm deep at most). The soft tissue must be retracted by the assistant during the bone cutting because any soft tissue will be pulled into the bur and stop it from revolving. It should be noted that the tooth, being basically sym-

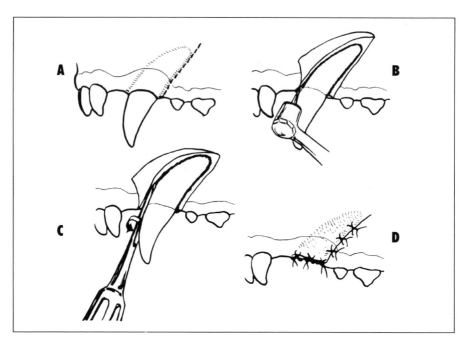

Figure 8-7

The upper canine of the dog must be extracted surgically unless it is seriously compromised with periodontitis.

(A) The first step is to incise from just caudal to the tooth to the root tip and then to elevate a flap of gingiva, mucosa, and periosteum.

(B) The tooth root is then outlined with the drill. Near the palatal edge, the trench around the tooth should be as deep as the tooth is wide, but farther apically just 1–2 mm of the cortical bone is cut.

(C) The elevator is inserted in the slot created on the rostral edge of the tooth and rotated to roll the tooth out of the alveolus.

(D) Mucosa and gingiva are sutured to complete the extraction.

metrical, is widest at the point above the CEJ where the palatal bone ends, so the troughs starting at the CEJ should flare before the root tapers. The entire root should be outlined.

Then the elevator is placed in the mesial trough along the tooth length, and with a twisting motion the tooth is rolled out of the alveolus, complete with the bone attached to its lateral surface. The gingiva is then sutured to cover the bone and alveolus that were exposed.

If the upper canine is mobile and/or an oronasal fistula already exists, the time spent on a surgical extraction is wasted, so the tooth is best elevated with the instrument placed rostrally and/or caudally only (to avoid further enlarging the fistula).

The lower canine of cats and dogs nearly always needs to be surgically extracted, unless there is severe periodontitis and the tooth is mobile. The problem here is that the tooth root is the major part of the thickness of the mandible, and forcing an elevator alongside the tooth can result in fracture of the bone supporting the lower incisors, the mandibular symphysis, or the rostral body of the mandible. (Note that before performing extractions on the mandible of a cat it is important to check whether the symphysis is already mobile. Many are not ossified but are only cartilaginous connections, and it is not sensible to take the blame for disarticulation if it was already present.)

To perform a surgical extraction of tooth 304 or 404 in either species, it is necessary first to sever the lateral frenulum, which ties the lower lip tight just caudal to the canine. In dogs the incision should be continued under the first premolar by leaving its attached gingiva intact and cutting at the MGL (mucogingival line). The root apex of the lower canine in the dog terminates medial to the area between the two roots of the second premolar, near another important structure—the mental foramen, the rostral termination of the mandibular canal. The rostral mandibular nerve and artery exit the canal at this point and should be protected from injury when elevating soft tissue or "burring" bone.

Unlike the upper canine, which is just under the cortical bone of the face, the root of the lower canine dives medial in the mandible. This means that thicker bone must be carved off of the tooth root to expose all of its lateral surface, which will allow its edges to be revealed and burred out for the final elevation. Happily, usually if the root is exposed only about half of its length, it tapers so dramatically that it can be moved by a medially placed elevator without applying undue pressure. If the tooth doesn't move, more apical bone is removed until it does.

Any other tooth may be extracted by "paintbrushing" off the cortical bone of either jaw followed by burring out a trough around the edges of the root(s). Of course, the soft tissues must first be elevated off of the bone in a mucoperiosteal flap, as in any surgical extraction. The upper fourth premolar presents more of a challenge than other premolars: although the buccal roots are readily available, the palatal root is not. However, once the buccal mesial root is removed, the bone between that root's alveolus and the palatal root can be burred away to reveal most of the palatal root. This tooth often has excess sharp bony projections that need to be removed (osteoplasty) to allow the gingiva and mucosa to be easily drawn over the extraction site and to make chewing more comfortable.

One tooth that is usually the culprit when extraction causes mandibular fracture is the lower first molar, or carnassial tooth. The roots (especially the mesial) of this tooth are very large and typically take up about 80 percent of the bulk of the jaw at this position. When periodontitis has destroyed much of the bone around one or both of these roots, elevation can cause a fracture very easily. To avoid fracture, and to prevent a long, arduous elevation in healthier bone, this tooth should be surgically extracted. Just as with the extraction of an upper carnassial, the lower molar extraction may uncover a projecting bone that needs to be contoured. To fill in bone in an extraction site more rapidly than it would if left to the natural process, cancellous bone grafts or synthetic bone matrices can be inserted into extraction sites (see Chap. 9).

TOOTH ATOMIZATION AND SUBGINGIVAL AMPUTATION

A confounding condition that arises in feline teeth is resorptive lesions in which significant portions of crown and root have been eaten away, leaving the remaining tooth structure dead and brittle. These often require surgical extractions. An alternative that sometimes may be used is "atomization" of roots. Except for the canine teeth, the roots of cat teeth are generally short enough that the root tip can be reached with the drill. When a crown snaps off during an attempt at elevation, atomization may be the best answer because digging with an elevator, especially in the mandible, can cause bone fracture. The bur is pushed gently down the root until resistance ceases as it "falls" through the bottom of the alveolus into cancellous bone or the mandibular canal. A light touch must be used because of the potential for damaging structures such as the mandibular artery. Once the bottom of the alveolus is reached, the bur is spiraled back out of the alveolus to remove the rest of the root. This is accomplished mainly by knowledge of the anatomy of the tooth and a sensitive touch (as soon as resistance is lost, the root is gone). A radiograph should reveal whether the entire root has been atomized.

Of course there are problems with this technique. The first is that the anatomy must be well understood before it is attempted, and the second is that deaths have been reported with root atomization in cats. The air that is blown into the tissues with a drill may cause an air embolus (when air bubbles get to the heart of a cat, the organ can "lose its prime," like a water pump).

Another method of extraction has been reported in cats and llamas but can be used in any animal. It involves amputating the tooth crown and distal root just below the gum line and suturing the gingiva to seal over it. The procedure must be done as aseptically as possible; a tooth compromised by periodontitis or endodontally is definitely not a good candidate (as, for instance, a stage 3 resorptive lesion). The advantage of subgingival amputation is that the alveolar crest is maintained, and the integrity of the jaw is not compromised, especially in those areas where the tooth root is a significant contributor to the strength of the bone (lower canine and carnassial teeth). There is no reason to treat the tooth pulp if the technique has been done relatively aseptically and a good seal is made with the sutured gingiva, but a pulp cap or root canal can also be performed (see Chap. 10). If the root is left in place, there will not be a loss of alveolar crest height.

AFTERCARE

Dental extractions can involve a great deal of pain for an animal, which should be addressed by the hospital. Chapter 6 contains techniques for administering local anesthetics and suggestions for postextraction analgesics (pain control). The comfort of patients should be a primary goal for veterinary staff, as it is for almost all owners. Owners appreciate and readily pay for pain control for their pets.

Assisting with Periodontics

Periodontitis is the most frequent cause of loss of teeth in dogs and cats. When it comes to periodontal care, the technician is usually in charge of ordinary prophies and root planing. The most frequent type of periodontal surgery is suturing of extraction sites, with or without osteoplasty and alveoloplasty, and this is covered in Chapter 8. Another area of surgery dealing with oral masses (usually cancer) is but briefly addressed in this chapter. The main thrust of this chapter is explaining surgical correction of periodontal lesions beyond simple root planing so that you can assist with such surgery.

The main tissue amenable to surgery is the gingiva, although bone sometimes is altered surgically. Periodontitis generally results in one of three outcomes: hyperplasia, recession, or pockets in the gingiva and other periodontal tissues (i.e., periodontal ligament and bone).

GINGIVOPLASTY

Many boxers display the characteristic tumorous-looking lesions of gingival hyperplasia, or hypertrophy, but it also occurs in other breeds of dog as well. It is rarely seen in cats. The condition apparently occurs when inflammation from oral microbes in plaque causes the stimulation of gingival growth (Fig. 9-1). The main increase in tissue is the fibrous subcutaneous component, although the epithelium responds as well to cover the increase in mass from underneath. At times the hypertrophied tissue is firmer than normal gingiva, while at others it seems to be essentially the same as normal. Occasionally there is extreme fibrosis and even partial calcification of the hypertrophied tissue, apparently due to long-term inflammation, but any sign that calcification has concurrently occurred in other tissues should be a clue to search for a systemic cause.

The extension of the gingiva over the crown creates what is known as a pseudopocket. Pseudopockets often occur in conjunction with true pocket development, where actual periodontal attachment loss occurs. In some dogs with gingival hyperplasia, the degree of gingival inflammation and plaque/calculus present does not seem to merit the reaction seen. Other affected dogs have copious calculus and extremely reddened gingiva. As long as there are pseudo- and true pockets, the inflammatory reaction will persist because the normal plaque-excluding function of the gingival sulcus is compromised. The swollen, distorted gingiva allows the incursion of plaque and calculus into the sulcus. The role of the veterinary dentist is

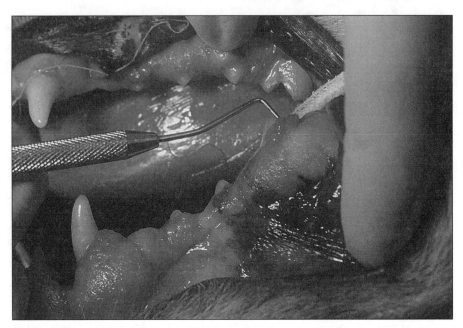

Figure 9-1

Gingival hyperplasia is a response to inflammation. Here the tissues have grown partially over the tooth crowns.

to cut off enough abnormal gingiva to restore the normal contour of the gingiva (gingivoplasty) and to combine this with thorough cleaning of the teeth to allow normal function to return.

There are several techniques for removing the extraneous tissue. Probably the most frequently used, because it is direct and the tools are most readily available, is simple sharp surgical excision—cutting it off with a scalpel blade. Because gingiva is very vascular, and because the inflamed gingiva is always even more vascular, there will be copious blood produced by the excisions. This makes the role of the assistant very important, to rinse away the blood with an air/water syringe or blot it with a gauze sponge so that surgery can proceed. Removing blood and water through suction (if available) is an additional service that is invaluable for the veterinarian performing the excisions.

To actually perform a gingivoplasty, very little is needed for equipment and supplies. There is the aforementioned air/water syringe and suction, gauze sponges, a cutting instrument, and a measuring instrument.

The actual depth of the sulcus must be measured because the free gingival margin of at least 2 mm must be maintained. Amputating the gingiva shorter will result in loss of attachment. The pocket marker is a clever little instrument that looks like a thumb forceps that exactly measures a 2-mm length. It has one blunt-edged flat piece that slides under the gingiva to the depth of the sulcus. The other side of the forceps has a sharp point, which when closed marks a pinpoint hole on the surface of the gingiva at the proper length. (In the absence of the forceps, a periodontal probe can be used to measure the depth of the hypertrophic gingiva, then placed on top of the gingiva to that length as a guide for how much to cut off.)

Then the scalpel (I prefer a size 15 blade) is used to make a beveled cut to the length of the markings. This is done to restore the normal, tapering edge of the gingiva. Although the surface will be raw and will tend to seep blood after the gingivoplasty, it will rapidly reepithelialize, and within a few days the gingiva will look normal. Cutting the extra gingiva off bluntly will perpetuate an abnormally thick gingiva, and hyperplasia will quickly recur. A disadvantage to sharp dissection is that the blade, which cuts the gingiva against the enamel surface, is rapidly dulled, and several may be required for one mouth.

There are other methods of cutting off the extra tissue. Some people prefer cautery. Cautery has the advantage of reducing the bleeding that occurs, but it has two disadvantages: Tissues take longer to heal than with surgical excision alone, and there is the potential for heat damaging periodontal structures and the tooth pulp if cautery is used clumsily. The wire loop is the least likely type of tip to cause such damage; it can be passed over the gingiva several times to "wipe away" the unwanted tissue. Compared with traditional cautery, radiocautery has the advantage of generating much less heat, but it has similar healing times. Radiocautery units are seldom seen in veterinary practices because they are so much more expensive than conventional cautery.

Another technique is the use of a dental drill with a finishing bur. The effect is somewhere between sharp excision and cautery. The drill has its own water supply and so would not require as much effort to remove blood from the surgical site. However, the bur would cause slight tearing and perhaps heat trauma to the gingiva. There is also some potential for surface damage to the tooth with the bur.

When animals treated for hyperplasia are sent home, it is wise to warn owners that they may see blood in the saliva for a day or two.

It is prudent to know what the animal's blood-clotting ability is before performing a gingivoplasty, especially if the patient is a dog that is a member of a breed subject to von Willebrand's disease. Any delay in clotting discovered when taking a blood sample or placing a catheter should be reported to the veterinarian.

GINGIVECTOMY AND OTHER "POCKET" SURGERIES

There are times when gingiva is amputated as a fast fix for periodontal pockets. When "normal" gingiva is amputated (that is, when gingiva positioned apically to the cemento-enamel junction [CEJ] is removed over a pocket) it is called a gingivectomy. Many times gingivoplasty is combined with gingivectomy because of pseudopockets and pockets coexisting in the same mouth. It is sometimes best to amputate gingiva if this will quickly return it to a smooth margin, but gingiva with the ability to attach to the bone should be maintained at all costs.

In the process of root planing a pocket, the curette naturally scrapes debris and epithelial tissues off of the soft tissue surface of the sulcus; this is called subgingival curettage. Ideally, this will be enough to allow the gingiva the chance to reattach to the bone (or tooth, if the alveolar bone is gone).

Sometimes, however, the epithelium of the gingiva has grown a thick layer to the depth of the pocket; as long as that layer of "outside" cells is present, the epidermal pegs will never attach down because fibroblasts in the subcutaneous tissues cannot push the epithelial cells out of the way. One way to treat this situation, if curettage is not adequate, is through a split-thickness gingivectomy: the thickness of the free gingival margin is split to the level of the sulcus, and the epithelium is removed that has formed next to the tooth.

A split-thickness gingivectomy is often combined with open root planing, where an incision is made on each side of the periodontal pocket wide enough that normal, functioning attached gingiva is included on each side. The flap is raised by scraping the gingiva off the bone to the depth of the pocket with a periosteal elevator or similar instrument. The root surface is then planed to smoothness and all necrotic debris removed, a split-thickness gingivectomy or subgingival curettage is performed to the level of healthy bleeding tissue, and the gingiva is replaced and sutured.

Apical repositioning of gingiva is a useful technique where there is significant recession and where a portion of attached gingiva appears marooned and doomed around an important tooth, such as a canine. The entire thickness of gingiva is raised, treated as above with curettage or a split-thickness gingivectomy, and then sutured farther toward the apex of the tooth root. This maintains the width of gingiva that might be lost with a simple gingivectomy to recontour edges.

Cautery should never be used for any surgery to maintain or salvage gingiva because too much tissue will be destroyed by heat; such surgery should be performed with sharp dissection only.

The role of the technician during these techniques is to retract and keep the surgical site clean after setting up the required instruments. Cutting suture ends will speed any surgery.

It will take a few days for attachment to begin to occur, and in that time the gingival surgery needs to be protected. A temporary collar of acrylic or composite restorative can be fashioned on the tooth so that food is deflected from the gingiva, and the animal can be given antibiotics to help support the tissues until they heal. In addition, home care of gentle lavage (rinsing or washing) with an antiseptic mouthwash (with a syringe or periodontal spray instrument such as a Waterpik) after the patient eats will also help maintain the periodontal surgery. It should be obvious that the dog should not be given bones, rawhides, or toys to gnaw during its convalescence or be allowed to play tug-of-war games that might damage the fragile surgery sites.

Home care is critical for periodontal surgery, and the tragedy is that people will pay for the surgeries—for themselves as well as their pets—and then not allow them to heal or forget about maintenance if they do heal. And then, of course, they blame the dentist for the failure.

ALVEOLOPLASTY, PERIODONTAL POCKET THERAPY, AND GUIDED TISSUE REGENERATION

Alveoloplasty

Alveolar bone must taper to the tooth for a healthy gingival attachment to form over it. When periodontitis has infected bone and caused it to necrose and its leading margin to recede, it may have a blunt termination after all necrotic debris has been cleaned off in open or closed root planing. This edge may be tapered with a cutting or general purpose bur to eliminate the void that would collect plaque and calculus if it were left untreated. When cutting bone, just as when cutting into a tooth that should not be damaged by heat, it is critical to have adequate water coolant to the bur. Otherwise, dead bone will result, which will create an even deeper pocket. Gingiva is sutured to cover an alveoloplasty as is done in the preceding surgeries.

Periodontal Pocket Therapy and Guided Tissue Regeneration

Once alveolar bone has been destroyed, it will not rebuild itself without a lot of help. The usual approach is to clean it thoroughly, ensure a tapered bony edge, and hope to salvage as much periodontal attachment as possible with essentially unaided natural healing.

A problem with healing is that the oral flora are still present and they may delay any attachment that might occur. One way to treat this is to give systemic antibiotics. However, despite the fact that the antibiotics are found in saliva and blood, they may not reach a high concentration in semidevitalized tissues in periodontal pockets. A way to get around this is to put antimicrobials into the pocket. To a certain extent we do this when we rinse the mouth with a substance like chlorhexidine after the prophy, but the effect is transient. Heska has developed a *perioceutic* (a coined term that combines "periodontal" and "therapeutic") to treat pockets. It contains an antibiotic combined with a carrier gel that becomes firm and attaches to soft tissues when placed in a cleaned periodontal pocket. The antibiotic action is intense locally, in the pocket where it is needed, for hours or days until the perioceutic falls out. Trials have shown that pocket depth can be reduced significantly with this product.

If an alveoloplasty won't leave enough bone for periodontal ligaments to attach it to a tooth, new bone and ligaments can be grown through guided tissue regeneration. To build up bone it is necessary (1) to provide a matrix on which the bone will grow and (2) to keep epithelium out. Some tissues simply proliferate faster than others. Of periodontal tissues, the slowest is bone, and the fastest is epithelium. Intermediate, but fairly fast, are the fibrocytes of the periodontal ligament. The bone needs the support of the periodontal ligament to attach it to the tooth.

If a bone matrix was implanted into a bony pocket and the epithelium of the gingiva simply sutured over it, the cells of the epithelium would divide rapidly to cover the bone matrix and essentially cover it over until epithelium reached the remaining periodontal ligament at the bottom of the pocket. Since the potential new bone would not be attached to the tooth by periodontal ligament, it would be absorbed by the body and lost. So the trick is to keep epithelium out until (1) the periodontal ligament fibrocytes can form new ligament to the tooth from the bottom of the pocket and (2) bone can be created and maintained. To do that, a membrane that excludes epithelium must be placed over the bone matrix and attached to the tooth at the level of desired depth of sulcus. The membrane material must be trimmed carefully to conform to the shape of the tooth and pocket in order to work properly.

The role of the technician in this process is to provide traction so that the veterinarian can see the surgery, to maintain as sterile a field as possible, and in many cases to mix dry artificial bone matrices with sterile saline or another source of fluid.

The use of autogenous (from the tissues of the same animal) bone grafts has a proven effectiveness but involves harvesting the cancellous bone graft material from a distant site aseptically and maintaining the graft material until the graft site is ready. Synthetic substitutes, although expensive, are much easier to use.

EXTRACTION SITE GRAFTS

Extraction sites sometimes make very large voids in the jaws. The blood clot that forms in an extraction site will first be infiltrated with fibrocytes, which will create a fibrous matrix for incoming osteocytes (bone cells). Eventually these bone cells will create irregular seams of bone that will finally fill in the entire defect. A way to speed the process is to deposit cancellous bone grafts or artificial bone matrix into the alveoli. These grafts need a clean (preferably aseptic) environment in which to thrive. Implanting the material into an extraction site filled with devitalized bone, infected granulomatous tissue, and other contaminated debris is an exercise doomed to failure, as epithelium over such a site will break down in the face of infection, losing the graft material as well as causing remaining graft material to be recycled by the body in a general cleanup effort.

One way to make a graft work is to wait until healing is well underway and the infection is under control. The extraction site is reopened two to eight weeks after the original extraction, and the graft placed. However, many clients want "one-stop shopping" and expect to have the graft placed in the same session as the extraction. This requires (1) that excavation of the extraction site—of dead bone and purulent and granulomatous tissue—be exacting, (2) that the site be thoroughly lavaged with disinfectant such as chlorhexidine, (3) that gingiva or mucosa sutured over the extraction site not be under tension or devitalized, and (4) that systemic antibiotics be administered for a period of at least two weeks after the procedure. Anything less than these precautions is inviting failure.

ORO-FACIAL SURGERY

There are several situations that are related to abnormal tooth or bone development or trauma that require surgery of the mandible or maxilla. Malplaced teeth can become impacted (be retained within the bone) and form a cystlike draining tract from the epithelial tissues trapped within the bone. A structure called a dentigerous cyst is a lost tooth structure that can be almost anywhere but is usually on the head. It may have a fully formed tooth, or portion of a tooth, within the fluid-filled structure. Other strange developmental abnormalities may mimic a tumor and cause distortion of oral structures because of growth. All of these types of structures may require excision (cutting them out) if they grow or cause problems because of size.

Trauma during development can cause teeth to grow in an abnormal position or fracture a bone in such a way as to cause it to lose its blood supply and become a sequestrum. Sequestra will develop a chronic draining tract and show areas of lysis in radiographs. They will not resolve by themselves because of the large area of bony tissue involved and so must be removed (fortunately, this is usually fairly easy to do because the margins of the dead tissue are so distinct and it doesn't bleed).

Congenital malformations, such as cleft palate/lip, periodontal pathology–induced oronasal fistulas (holes between the mouth and nasal passages, usually at the level of the canine tooth), and traumatic injuries to palate or lips, may require flap surgery to close deficits. The soft tissue flaps must be treated with care if they are to be successful. Most notably they should not be sutured under tension. Oral malignancies (cancer) often require bone as well as soft tissue surgery.

Bleeding and an obstructed view are the most common problems in most surgeries involving the mouth. Stabilization of the head is another. Especially when a reciprocating bone saw is used, it may be very difficult to keep the head steady. It may mean using several layers of tape pierced by the canine teeth to pull the jaws open and attaching the tape to the table. Veterinary dentists tend to prefer the use of a dental drill with cutting bur to a bone saw, which is what orthopedic (bone) surgeons usually use.

The most common type of oral malignancy in the dog is the malignant melanoma; by far the most common in the cat is the squamous cell carcinoma. The first surgery that is usually performed on any oral malignancy is a biopsy, either excisional (with the presumption that all of the visible tumor will be taken off) or incisional (only a sample of the tumor will be taken) for histology. Microscopic examination will then reveal the type of tumor (Fig. 9-2). When a tumor invades bone or comes from a bone source (osteosarcoma or chondrosarcoma, from bone and cartilage, respectively), the biopsy may be restricted to the soft tissue component, or a piece of the abnormal mineralized tissue may be submitted. The histological (microscopic) diagnosis will provide a prognosis (what is likely to happen) and direct the course of action. Since most of the oral malignancies invade bone, removal of the tumor is going to involve removal of part of the mandible or maxilla, and since a generous margin must be maintained, it may well be a large and disfiguring portion of the face. Surgery on oral and facial malignancies must be aggressive to have a chance at a cure.

The armamentarium of equipment for oro-facial surgery includes all of the instruments that are needed for general soft tissue surgery as well as those for

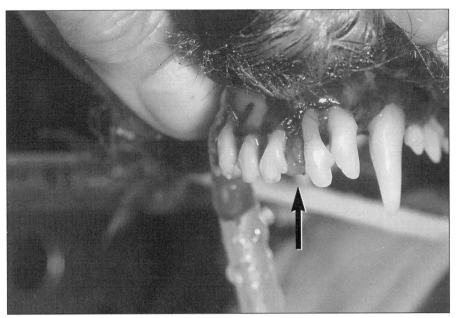

Figure 9-2

Oral tumors (*arrow*) are often grossly distinguishable from hypertrophic gingiva by the absence of periodontal inflammation, absence of multiple lesions, surface characteristics that differ from gingiva (color, texture, etc.), and areas of necrosis or involvement with bone (destruction and/or proliferation). A biopsy is the only way to tell for sure.

bone surgery. Bone saws, whether hand or air powered, are used, obviously, to cut through the bone. Osteotomes (bone chisels) and a mallet are necessary to cut through remaining bone tissue after the main cuts are made. Cautery is a necessity for bone surgery of the face; bleeders tend to be profuse, and when vessels are cut by the saw, they tend to retract into the bone, where they cannot be caught and ligated readily. Soft tissue must be elevated off bone before cutting, requiring periosteal elevators.

The assistant, in addition to readying instruments, will be required to steady the head if there is movement and to retract tissues with a Senn or other type of tissue retractor. It may also be necessary to make blood transfusions in instances of profuse blood loss, for which the potential exists whenever significant portions of either jaw are removed.

There is a method of painting the edges of the tissue removed with India ink so that the histologist can determine where the actual cut edge of the material is (as opposed to an artificial edge that may occur during processing). This job usually falls to the technician because the surgeon is busy closing the surgical site.

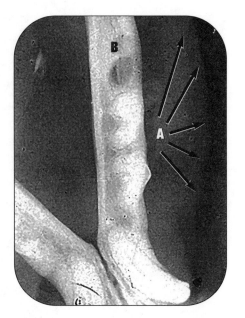

Figure 9-3

The firm mass (A) on the side of this cat's mandible was not continuous with the bone, as shown in the X ray. The diagnosis was complicated by severe periodontitis around the first molar, which was extracted before the X ray was taken (*see dark area*, B).

In general, for surgery to be curative of virtually any cancer, generous allowances around the tumor material are needed to ensure "clean" margins (edges); if there are cancerous cells that escape removal, the tumor will recur. Knowing the extent of the tumor is the key. This is determined by gross appearance and, when bone is involved, by X ray (Fig. 9-3). Unfortunately, many oral tumors are not found until they are quite large or have spread locally or systemically (through the rest of the body).

Some of these oro-facial surgeries can be very painful, and use of local or regional nerve blocks is important (Chap. 6). Also, the provision of long-term analgesia, such as that found in fentanyl patches, should be mandatory. Following the surgery the technician assists with the aftercare of the patient.

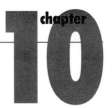
Assisting with Endodontics

Therapy to the tooth pulp—endodontics—involves three basic procedures: the root canal, apexification, and the pulp cap. These are always performed by the veterinarian, but assistance by the technician—readying tools and supplies and taking radiographs—immeasurably speeds any of these procedures. The root canal, which is the best known because of its frequency in human dentistry, is a salvage operation for a tooth with a dead pulp in which all infected pulp is removed and is replaced by a combination of inert and bacteriostatic or bacteriocidic materials. A surgical root canal, or apicoectomy, is the same thing except that in addition to filling the pulp chamber the apex of the root is also sealed. The apexification procedure is used when a tooth is dead but is too immature to have a complete apex to the root. This pulp chamber is cleaned out and filled with calcium hydroxide, which allows the root tip to form. Finally, the pulp cap, or vital pulpotomy, is an effort to save the life of a tooth pulp that has been exposed to the mouth due to trauma or crown amputation. The root canal and apexification are procedures that a veterinarian needs to perform frequently in order to stay proficient; the pulp cap is a much less technically demanding procedure that any practice should be able to offer.

THE ROOT CANAL

Indications for Use

To many people, the root canal seems to be a defining feature of dental practice. How often, when mention is made of dental services, do we hear "And do you do root canals and everything?" The root canal definitely is a valuable therapy. It obliterates infected or dead pulp and seals the tooth from the bone to prevent the tooth being the source of bacteria for apical infection in the bone.

Many people have experienced the agony of an abscessed tooth. In humans, probably because of the open canal shape of the root apex (as opposed to the nearly closed, delta shape in most dogs and cats) and probably due to differences in circulating bacteria and susceptibility to them, abscessed teeth usually occur without exposure of the pulp to oral microorganisms; in other words, the teeth are not fractured. These abscesses occur because of a condition called anachoresis, which starts with an area of tissue that is inflamed for whatever reason (as in trauma). When this anachoretic area happens to be a tooth pulp, bacteria in the bloodstream find a congenial home in the inflamed tissue and colonize it. The multiplying bacteria cause the liberation of tissue substances (kinins) that initiate more inflammation and attract white blood cells, which become pus. When this sequence occurs within bone, the pressure causes death of the tissues and intense pain. When the dentist opens the abscess, pus pours out, and the person often feels immediate release.

Horses also have open apical canals, so apparently they too can suffer from anachoretic abscessation, in which teeth will abscess without pulp exposure to the mouth. It probably occurs to a much lesser degree in dogs and cats; the proof of this is that it is very rare to see evidence of apical abscessation on survey radiographs of teeth with unbroken crowns.

Internal abscesses eventually find a way to drain by dissolving tissue until pus can flow out of the body in a draining tract. Tooth abscesses may drain several different directions according to where the root is located. They may flow into the mouth, into the nose, or out of the skin of the face or lower jaw. If they are continuous with periodontal pockets, they are combination perioendo abscesses and drain out beside the tooth. Abscess tracts in the mouth that do not drain periodontally, which are the majority, usually appear as an ulcer at the mucogingival junction.

In dogs and cats, the usual initiation of an apical abscess is a fractured tooth. Bacteria in the mouth first contaminate the tooth pulp at the exposure site. Then, if nothing is done to prevent it (like administering antibiotics or a performing a pulp cap), the bacteria multiply and set up an inflammatory response, called pulpitis, in the tooth pulp chamber. Pulpitis is very uncomfortable because it involves swelling within a rigid space. Eventually the tooth pulp dies, and infection reaches the apical bone and results in an apical abscess. This process takes variable amounts of time because of differences in bacteria (numbers and type) and in the ability of the body to fight off infection. For instance, if a young dog has an infected pulp that is large and has a great blood supply, this dog may fight off infection longer than an older one with an infected pulp that has a limited blood supply. In radiographs (Fig. 10-1), an apical abscess appears as a dark area around the apex of the tooth (or as *radiolucent*, meaning that the X rays passed through the lack of bone to expose the film).

The period in which the tooth is most sensitive (when pulpitis is active before the pulp dies and when the apical abscess is forming before it finds a way to drain) is often missed by owners and veterinarians alike. The animal's teeth can be tapped as a test: A simple tap on the tooth with the open fracture will usually make the animal flinch. If the tooth is painful, but is dead, root canal therapy or an extraction should be performed. Antibiotics are only palliative; they will only temporarily eliminate infection while they clean up bacteria that can be reached by the blood supply. The bacteria in the dead tissue of the pulp live to thrive another day.

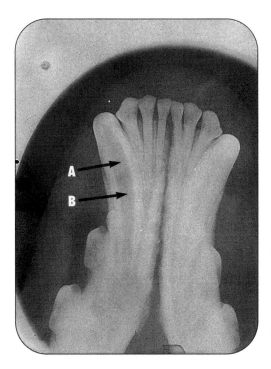

Figure 10-1

A fractured tooth (A) with an apical root abscess (the dark area at the apex of the root, B). Note how wide the canal of this tooth is compared with the other canine. This tooth was fractured, and the pulp died due to infection. The apex of the tooth never closed off.

Many animals respond to infection at the root apex by mobilizing bone cells to wall off the abscess. This bone tends to ankylose (fuse) the root tip to the bone. If the bone seal is effective, the animal may show no sign of pain. However, there is always the potential for bacteria to break through. Abscesses that grow over a long period of time release bacteria into the bloodstream constantly and have been shown to seed bacteria hematogenously (through the bloodstream) to distant organs. Therefore, it is best not to ignore old open fractures; the effect on the animal may be subtle but significant.

The root canal may be performed in the presence of an abscess unless there has been significant internal or external resorption of the root of the tooth. Slight resorption at the apex can be dealt with by an apicoectomy, which includes sealing the apex.

The equipment and materials for root canals (which are explained in more detail later) are simple: dental burs for entry into the canal or expansion, barbed broaches to capture and pull out devitalized pulp (if it is intact), files and reamers to clean the canal, a solvent/lubricant preparation for filing, a disinfecting solution and syringes and needles for use after filing, paper points

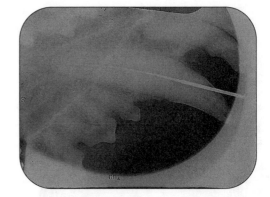

Figure 10-2
X ray of tooth with a file in the canal.

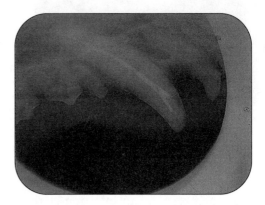

Figure 10-3
X ray of a filled canal.

to remove remaining solution, gutta percha points to fill the canal, endodontal forceps for placing paper and gutta percha points, spreaders and pluggers to work the gutta percha, cement to fill in around the gutta percha, and finally, materials and equipment for the final restoration.

Root canal therapy relies heavily on radiology; a root canal should never be attempted without the use of X rays. There are a minimum of four X rays that should be taken for a root canal: the assessment radiograph, to ensure that there is adequate root structure to seal with a root canal; the largest file that will reach the tip of the pulp cavity (Fig. 10-2), to demonstrate that the full length of the canal has been instrumented; the first gutta percha point ("master point") in the canal, to show that it goes to the apex of the canal; and the final fill, to show that it completely obliterates space, especially at the apex (Fig. 10-3). In reality, most veterinarians take more than this minimum because often a radiograph shows that the desired effect has not been met (the file does not go to the apex, etc.).

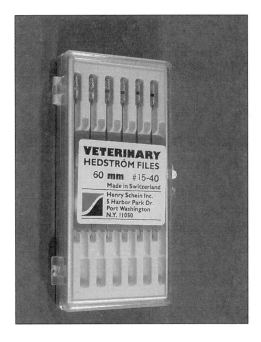

Figure 10-4

Hedstrom files are one type of file used to remove soft, infected tissue from the pulp chamber.

The Procedure

Once the assessment X ray has been taken, the veterinarian must create access to the pulp chamber. Depending on the tooth, the number of roots, and the degree of curve of the affected root, he or she may decide to make one or more access sites to the pulp chamber. The usual bur to make access is a round or pear-shaped bur, the size depending on the minimum diameter needed to fit files into the canal. It is critical not to take excessive tooth structure away because all restoratives (fillings) are weaker than the tooth or weaken the tooth by being too large and causing the surrounding tooth structure to break with pressure. A special flexible bur, the Gates-Glidden, is sometimes used to enlarge the access hole.

Barbed broaches are disposable metal instruments that have tiny hairlike curved arms that act like the barbs of cockleburs or other annoying burs in nature; they are meant to catch onto tissue. They are useful only if the pulp has not liquified due to long-term infection. They are inserted into the canal, twisted, and pulled out; ideally, the entire pulp will come out in one piece with the broach because this makes the rest of the instrumentation of the canal very easy. However, this is seldom the case.

Any remaining soft tissue pulp content and any dentin that has been degraded by infection must be cleaned out before the final filling of the canal can progress. This is done with the use of endodontal files. The twisted, tapering files come in two types, Hedstrom (Fig. 10-4) and K-files. They have slightly

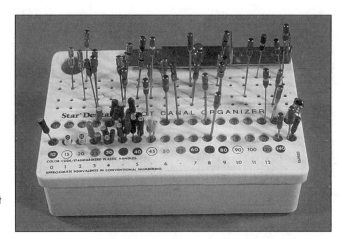

Figure 10-5

A file organizer keeps the different-sized files readily at hand in a disinfectant bath.

different cross sections, although both have cutting edges that engage when they are pulled out, rather than when they are inserted. K-files have an advantage in that they can be screwed into the dentin and then withdrawn; if this is done with a Hedstrom file, it will usually break or at least unwind its twist. Hedstrom files are used only with an in-and-out motion. Another filelike instrument that is frequently used to enlarge the canal quickly in the distal portion is the reamer. It has flutes like the K-file but about half as many turns, and it is relatively strong and cuts very efficiently.

Files come in different lengths and widths. The two standard lengths for veterinary dentistry are the short (35 mm) length that is used in human dentistry and the long (55 mm) that is useful for large canine teeth in dogs, which have roots much too long for the human files. The files vary from size 10, which is as fine as a human hair, to the approximate size of pencil lead. The files all have the same degree of taper and are sized according to diameter at a certain length from the tip (16 mm). Reamers are intermediate in length between the two file sizes and are sized by diameter as well. Clean files are best stored in a file organizer (Fig. 10-5), which has holes for the proper size of files, a sponge body to hold the files in place, and a container to fill and saturate the sponge with disinfectant solution. After the files have been used, they are most easily kept in a small sponge holder because they are small and easy to lose or bend during cleanup (the pointed ends are also exceptionally sharp and can cause painful, contaminated puncture wounds).

Preferences vary, but the canals are generally filed in a "step-down" technique, with the smallest files used first to get to the tip of the apex, followed with larger and larger files as the canal gets wider. A small file is usually utilized at the end "to recapitulate"—that is, to drag out any filings that may

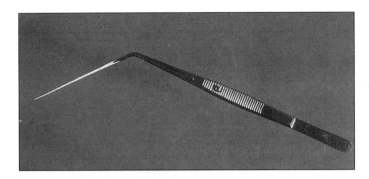

Figure 10-6

An endodontal forceps holding a paper point. Paper points are used to dry the canal after disinfection.

have been pushed to the apex during the larger file use. The canal is filed until only clean, white shavings of white dentin are retrieved. A solvent/lubricant solution is often used to aid in the filing process, but it is not absolutely necessary. When the canal is presumed to be fully filed, or "instrumented," the largest file that reaches the farthest into the canal is placed, and a radiograph taken. If the file goes to the end of the apical canal, the process can continue; if it is shorter, further filing is necessary, or a smaller file must be used.

The canal must be disinfected to remove the majority of residual bacteria. The usual disinfecting solution is sodium hypochlorite—common household bleach—diluted 50 percent as it comes out of the bottle (i.e., diluted to 2.625 percent sodium hypochlorite). It is instilled by syringe with a 22 g hypodermic needle or a special endodontal needle. It is very important not to push the needle so that it forms a seal in the canal, as the bleach can be forced through the apex of the tooth into the bone, which will cause a painful necrosis. Another disinfecting solution that can be used is 1–2 percent chlorhexidine gluconate or diacetate. Neither will cause the severe reaction in the bone, and each is probably preferable to sodium hypochlorite in cases in which the apex may be an open canal. No matter which disinfectant is used, it is dispensed near the apex of the root and allowed to flush the canal thoroughly. Excess bleach should be absorbed with gauze sponges as it exits the tooth and immediately rinsed off of any oral tissues it contacts.

After disinfecting the canal, the remaining solution must be removed before the canal is filled. This is done with absorbent paper points (Fig. 10-6). The veterinarian will call for paper points the same size as the canal, and as the technician, you will hand them over, held in endodontal forceps. You need to be sure to handle the points only with the forceps and only on the widest end; the paper points come sterile, and touching the fine tips with your fingers or

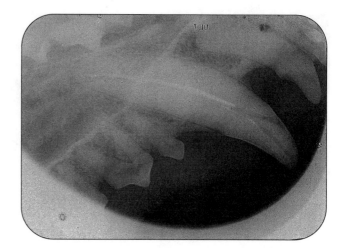

Figure 10-7

An X ray is taken after the first (master) point is placed in the canal to make sure that it obturates (fills) the root apex.

endodontal instrument will introduce bacteria into the disinfected canal. You should have a loaded forceps ready when the veterinarian reaches for it (in other words, you need to stay one or two steps ahead of the veterinarian). The larger the canal, the more paper points will be needed. When a paper point comes out of the canal dry, it is time for the gutta-percha fill.

Gutta percha is a natural latex-type material that comes from the sap of a tree, similar to the material from rubber trees that used to be our only source of rubber (before rubber was artificially synthesized). Gutta percha does not support the growth of bacteria, so it is functionally inert as far as infections go. By tradition gutta percha is usually tinted pink, but there is gutta percha available in multiple colors by size (width). The gutta percha "points" are all rolled to a taper and vary from a hair's thickness to about that of a thick pencil lead. There are regular (human) lengths of about 35 mm and "veterinary" lengths of about 60 mm to fill the long canals of large dogs' canine teeth. The veterinarian selects a size of gutta percha point that he or she thinks will fit exactly into the apex of the canal according to the size of the largest file that reached the apex. This is the master point. If it is short of the apex on the X ray (Fig. 10-7), a smaller point is chosen, or the apex is reinstrumented because there is probably debris in the apex. The gutta percha point is handled in a similar way to the paper point; the veterinarian will indicate what size is desired.

If the master point is satisfactorily filling the apex, it is removed, and it or another the same size is coated with cement. The cement used for root canals may be simply a combination of zinc oxide powder and eugenol (oil of cloves), or it may contain barium (which has the advantage of being radiopaque on an

X ray) or other substances. Both zinc oxide and eugenol inactivate bacteria. Whatever cement is used, it will eventually harden in the tooth and fill any voids around the gutta percha. The technician has the job of preparing the endodontal cement by spatulating drops of oil into the powder. Preparation of the cement is done with a spatula on a glass slab; the process of spatulation is to scrape the materials together with the edge of the spatula and then to squish them together with the flat blade repeatedly. Stirring is ineffective. There are different preferences for thickness of the material, from heavy cream to a stiff paste. The main thing is that it must be consistent and have no areas of heavier powder or more oil in one part than another.

Most of the time the gutta percha points are merely coated in the cement before they are inserted, but some veterinarians like to fill the canal with cement before inserting points. This is done either with a spiro-lentula filler (a special, fine spiral instrument) on a slow-speed handpiece or with a clean endofile. The veterinarian indicates the size and approximate numbers of points expected to be used, and the technician makes them available in forceps as they are needed. (Unused points can be reinserted into their containers to use another time if they are not touched or their fragile points bent.) Between insertion of the points the veterinarian melts off the ends of the gutta percha outside the tooth with cautery (a special endodontal heating element) or an instrument flamed to adequate heat to melt the material. Gutta percha, being a rubberlike material, does not cut cleanly except with heat. Usually, after each piece of gutta percha is inserted, a spreader is inserted into the canal to push all other points aside to make a space for the next point. Heated spreaders make the process easier but can pull gutta percha out by melting it to the instrument. Another instrument, the plugger, has a blunt end and is used to force gutta percha apically. An intermediate X ray may be used to see if the fill of the canal is proceeding according to plan.

When the fill is complete, the gutta percha should be a few millimeters from the surface of the tooth. An intermediate restorative material that is compatible with eugenol can be placed, or the final restorative placed over the gutta percha after proper preparation (see Chap. 11). The final fill of a root canal should be x-rayed to ensure that the entire length of the pulp chamber has been filled (Fig. 10-8).

To visualize what a root canal can do to strengthen a tooth, imagine a drinking straw with liquid within it (as in liquified, necrotic pulp in a tooth). The top of the straw is open (into the bone, if this were a tooth). The straw will bend readily if any force is applied to it, as will a tooth, except that the tooth wall fractures. Now imagine that liquid rubber has been poured into the straw and has become solid. The straw will not readily bend. The added advantage for the tooth is that the cement that is used will not support the growth of bacteria, and any apical infection can be cleaned up by antibiotics or the body's own defenses.

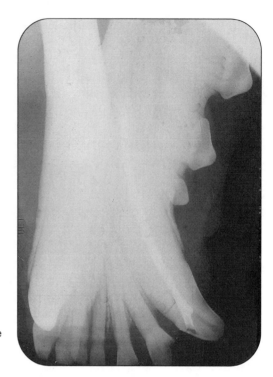

Figure 10-8
The final fill of a root canal should also be x-rayed to make sure that the entire length of the pulp chamber has been filled.

Apicoectomy: The Surgical Root Canal

Occasionally a root canal fails; usually this is because of inadequate fill at the apex of the root. To correct the situation, an apicoectomy (apical obturation) must be performed: the access of bacteria from the tooth into the bone must be eliminated, so the root apex is amputated and a restoration placed in it to plug the end of the tooth. An X ray will indicate the apical lucency (radiolucency) of an abscess.

A flap of mucosa over the root (or roots, in a multirooted tooth in which more than one has abscessed) is lifted to expose the bone, and a cutting bur used to expose the root tip. The tooth is then opened with a beveled cut to reveal all edges of the root tip, and the apical 2 or more millimeters of the canal cleaned out.

Several restoratives can be used to obturate the apex; amalgam may be used or one of several intermediate restoratives. These last have the advantage of forming an attachment to the tooth surface, whereas amalgam must be packed into place. Amalgam often leaves radiodense particles around the tooth; the material is crumbly until packed, and pieces tend to get away and they may be hard to find.

The devitalized bone around the tooth apex must be scraped out with excavators until only vital, dense bone remains. A variety of methods may be used if the site of the root apex becomes contaminated by blood from the bone before it can be obturated.

The bone may be packed with cotton pellets with or without a coagulant such as calcium hydroxide, or the cotton may be soaked in epinephrine, which causes spasm of small blood vessels (epinephrine should never be used if the animal is on halothane gas). Cotton pellets should always be counted so that they can be retrieved because leaving a foreign material in the abscess site is certain to cause another abscess. The technician is the one who should keep the count, when handing the cotton pellets to the veterinarian and as they are retrieved. Coagulants that cause tissue necrosis, like silver nitrate, should not be used. Judicious use of electrocoagulation is acceptable.

The abscess site should be flushed with a solution of a disinfectant such as povidone-iodine or chlorhexidine before it is closed. A blood clot will form in the abscess site, which will eventually fill in with bone. The mucosa is closed with an absorbable suture.

APEXIFICATION

When a young tooth suffers an open fracture, the inevitable result is an apical abscess. This is because the infection in the tooth covers a large area of bone—just as if a large shard of bone lost its blood supply and became an infected sequestrum (see Chap. 8 for how a tooth root can become a sequestrum). For the most part, the periodontal ligament is alive and well and protects the infected tooth from invasion by blood vessels and phagocytic white blood cells, except for the area of the open apex. The bone cannot wall off that large an infection. And so we get a draining abscess.

The usual tooth to suffer from an immature tooth fracture and abscess is the canine because the root apex does not form until the dog (or cat) is 14 to 18 months old. The tooth root, at this stage, is a thin shell at the apical end, with the dentin thicker in the crown (but with the pulp chamber still very wide). The first thing that must be done is to instrument the dead, necrotic pulp out of the tooth. This is essentially the same process as that of the root canal, except that it is much more exacting. There is a much larger space to clean out, and since the wall is very thin, care must be taken not to perforate it because a seal would be impossible in the root canal that would follow apexification.

The goal of apexification is to induce the tooth to finish apexifying the tip of the root. This will take variable amounts of time according to how old the tooth was when it died and how viable Hertwig's epithelial root sheath is. The cells of the sheath, which are responsible for determination of the root growth, are amazingly resilient, and even when pulp is dead, they can carry on once the infection is removed.

The empty pulp chamber is flushed to remove as much soft tissue debris as possible before filling it with a substance congenial to bone. A disinfectant like dilute Betadine or chlorhexidine is preferable to sodium hypochlorite because of the negative (sometimes dramatic) reaction of the bone to the bleach.

The pulp chamber is completely filled with calcium hydroxide. In order to make the calcium hydroxide radiopaque, 10 percent barium sulfate is added to the calcium and mixed thoroughly. The calcium hydroxide is basic and potentially irritating to tissues, like skin, but bone can thrive in its presence. Bacteria, on the other hand, cannot live in it. In fact, the calcium provides one of the building blocks of the new dentin that is needed to form the apex of the tooth while protecting the bone from further infection.

Placement of the calcium hydroxide is tedious. The powder may be made into a thick paste by mixing with water or saline, or it may be used in its powder form. Either way, it is usually placed in the tooth by means of amalgam carriers or a dental syringe (for paste only). The technician fills the amalgam carrier or syringe tip by packing the calcium mixture into it and handing the filled instrument to the veterinarian. Either method is going to require numerous loads of calcium hydroxide followed by tamping with an endodontal plugger. The entire pulp chamber is filled with the calcium mixture, and a restoration (or more than one if a second access site has been made) is placed over the calcium. Use of a calcium hydroxide cement will aid in placing the final restoration because it forms a solid base for the "filling." Complete filling of the pulp chamber is verified by X ray.

Apexification is only step one of the procedure. In humans, the calcium hydroxide dressing is changed every month or two until the tooth apexifies, but in cats and dogs the first is usually the only dressing until the apex closes. At that time the calcium hydroxide is removed, and a conventional (except that it means filling a huge pulp chamber) root canal is performed to strengthen the tooth. The calcium mixture tends to be absorbed by the blood supply as the tooth forms an apex, and the tooth is therefore mainly filled with fluid and some calcium, which has little strength.

THE PULP CAP

Probably the most valuable endodontal service a hospital can provide is the pulp cap. This procedure is also known as a vital pulpotomy and a direct pulp cap. Essentially it is used on a fractured tooth to seal off the pulp from the mouth with a restoration while dressing the pulp with a congenial substance of—what else?—calcium hydroxide. The process not only usually saves the life of the tooth and eliminates infection but it also immediately removes the pain of an open pulp and exposed nerve for the animal. Many cats with a tooth fracture caused by trauma refuse to eat until the tooth is sealed. This behavior, of course, is counterproductive to healing in general because adequate nutrition is necessary for bodily repair. Dogs usually show the pain by drooling, aversion to pulling games, or aversion to drinking cold water, but many show no apparent sign, which is why root canals are necessary later!

The pulp cap generally must be performed within 24 to 48 hours after the injury, although there are exceptions to the rule. Usually the sooner after trauma (preferably within a very few hours), the greater the chance of success. Bacteria need several hours to colonize the pulp, although in filthy mouths there would be a larger bacterial burden to start with, and it would then progress more rapidly. A pulp that has a good blood supply would be expected to be more able to control infection than one with a compromised blood supply.

A pulp that will bleed when the clot is removed and which has a firm history of very recent fracture should be a good candidate for a pulp cap, but time is of the essence. The fresh fracture is a dental emergency. It can be delayed if the animal is placed on antibiotics for a day or two if there is no way to perform the pulp cap, but the longer the wait, the more likely that bacteria will kill the pulp.

The equipment and supplies needed for a pulp cap are minimal. If the tooth has a highly angled fracture, it must be amputated (with a cutting or general purpose bur) so a table of dentin is available in which to place a restoration after the pulp is treated. A sterile round or pear-shaped bur is a necessity. After the tooth has been cleaned and disinfected with chlorhexidine or povidone-iodine, the bur is put on the handpiece without contaminating the tip after any water in the handpiece line is evacuated by running it dry (with another bur or a blank). The sterile bur is used dry because water in the unit would most likely contain some bacteria; the bur is used for such a short time that it will not generate heat.

The bur, which is chosen for the minimum size needed to create an opening in the coronal canal for an instrument, is passed quickly into and out of the canal from 4 to 10 mm deep. This tears and amputates the soft tissue in the distal canal and is the reason the procedure is called a vital pulpotomy; live but contaminated pulp is removed so that a dressing of calcium hydroxide can be placed over the remaining pulp.

The next task is to place calcium hydroxide powder on the pulp. Occasionally the pulp will bleed excessively, and powder will be rapidly washed away. Some way needs to be found to make the pulp stop bleeding without harming it. The best thing to do this with is the calcium hydroxide itself, with light pressure. A sterile paper point is either inserted butt first into the canal or cut off aseptically, wetted with sterile saline, and passed through the calcium hydroxide powder until the powder clings to the end of the point; this is then placed into the tooth in light contact with the bleeding tissue for up to a minute or two. The process can be repeated if bleeding results in a washout of the powder. Slight bleeding causes no problems, but the absence of bleeding may indicate that, rather than being fresh, the fracture is old and the tooth is nonvital.

The calcium hydroxide is gently packed a minimum of 2 mm over the pulp. The easiest way to deliver the calcium hydroxide to the tooth is to pack it into amalgam carriers, which are discharged into the pulp chamber, and then to lightly tamp it into contact with the pulp with a plugger; the technician can hand the loaded amalgam carriers to the veterinarian as he or she needs them. The calcium hydroxide gives the pulp an adequate insulation, provides calcium to build more dentin, and irritates the pulp just enough to stimulate the mobilization of odontoblasts to build a dentinal bridge under the restoration that will be placed over the dressing.

An intermediate restoration material, such as a calcium hydroxide cement, may be placed over the calcium hydroxide powder in order to have a firm foundation for the final restoration (the technician, of course, is useful here to mix the cement as it is needed). However, some final restorations can be placed directly atop the powder. It is important that the calcium hydroxide powder not have barium in it and that the restoration not be radiopaque either because follow-up radiographs must show the wispy, radiolucent dentinal bridge, the formation of which is the object of the procedure. Amalgam should not be used: it is strongly radiopaque. Deep restorations are necessary in a dog that is abusive to its teeth, but a restoration may be as shallow as 2 mm and still seal the pulp adequately. (See Chap. 11 for information about restorations.)

Radiographs are necessary as a follow-up to ensure that the tooth is alive and that the tooth is not abscessing. In a young dog or cat, the cessation of narrowing of the canal will tell you that the tooth has died. A dead tooth may also be identified by transillumination with a strong light source; dead teeth are less translucent than live teeth (they usually look remarkably

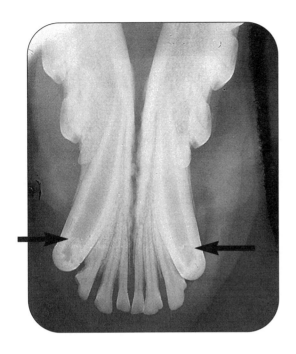

Figure 10-9

A successful pulp cap will show the presence of a dentinal bridge, where the odontoblasts have sealed off the pulp chamber under the restoration with new dentin. It is important to use a nonradiopaque restorative to show the dentinal bridge. This dog had bilateral crown amputations with pulp caps of the lower canines as therapy for teeth that were striking the palate. At four months postpulp cap, both teeth are showing the development of dentinal bridging under the restorations (see arrows).

chalky). The tooth should be radiographed at least four to six months after the pulp cap to visualize the dentinal bridge (Fig. 10-9). If the dentinal bridge is absent, the tooth may be dead. The best therapy for a dead tooth is a root canal.

To make sure there is no other pulpal pathology, at least one X ray before the pulp cap is prudent, although not always necessary if the fracture is definitely fresh and the tooth is solidly rooted. If the tooth is loose, it could mean that it is fractured just under the gingiva, where you can't see it. This tooth is doomed. However, a root tip fracture without contamination can heal quite nicely, although there may be root resorption in the future.

Endodontic therapy is an integral part of the complete dental service. To preserve the life of a tooth or to maintain a tooth in the mouth for function and appearance while relieving active or chronic infection provides benefit to the animal, the owner, and the hospital.

Assisting with Orthodontics, Prosthodontics, and Restorative Dentistry

The topics in this chapter are grouped together for the simple reason that they all involve, among other things, the improvement of the appearance of the teeth. As a matter of definition, orthodontics involves moving the teeth (*dontics*) around in the bone until they are straight (*ortho*) when there is a malocclusion (when the teeth meet incorrectly). Prosthodontics involves replacements for teeth, like prosthetic limbs; the most common—albeit rather rare—type of prosthodontics for pets is a full crown. Dental restoratives are substances that restore the teeth in appearance and/or function, such as "fillings" for root canals or caries.

The technician can be invaluable for the smooth, efficient performance of orthodontics, prosthodontics, and restorative dentistry. In some cases you may be asked only to get materials and instruments ready for use and to clean them up; in others, to make models and impressions as certain dental hygienists do.

ORTHODONTICS

It is extremely rare to perform orthodontics on cats, but the principles are essentially the same as for a small dog. Most breeds of dogs have a variation from the "wild" type of dentition because selective breeding has altered the head shape to fit a breed standard. Some of the breed standards of tooth occlusion are poorly functional, such as those for the brachycephalic (short-faced) bulldog and pug. In these breeds, the face is short, but the mandible stays essentially a normal length. The teeth do not interdigitate normally, and the result is that the teeth are not very efficient in chewing food or cleaning themselves during the chewing of fibrous, fleshy foods. Other breeds have less obvious deviations from normal. In many of the small or toy breeds, teeth have not miniaturized as much as the jaws, and the result can be crowding. In addition, many of these dogs are subject to retained deciduous ("baby") teeth, which exacerbates the crowding in the mouth. There are certain breeds in which a shorter, blockier face has become more stylish, and breeders have chosen animals that show a shorter nose, without taking into account that they are selecting for a shorter upper jaw (maxilla) while ignoring the mandible. This has resulted in the mandible essentially staying the same length as in the ancestors, while the maxilla shortens. The obvious result is a type III malocclusion, or an apparently protruding lower jaw (although, in actuality, the mandible is fine—it is the maxilla that has changed). Although there are no breeds in which the lower incisors are supposed to be in front of the upper incisors, except for the brachycephalics (the bulldog, pug, etc.), a survey of breed standards will reveal breeds for which a level bite as well as a scissors bite of the incisors and canines are acceptable. These are breeds that

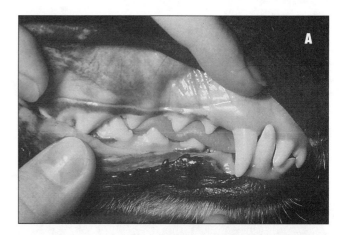

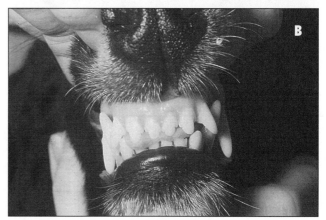

Figure 11-1

A dog that has a good bite.

(A) Lateral view. Note that the lower canine is equidistant between the upper canine and the upper third incisor. Also, look at the zigzag (or pinking shears) orientation of the premolars. The tip of each premolar "points" to the space between the premolars in the opposite jaw.

(B) Rostral view. The upper incisors are just rostral to the lowers, and the midline of each jaw is lined up.

have been genetically manipulated for a shorter face. Other breeds, particularly those that have been bred for long heads, are subject to problems due to a very short lower jaw. Certain breeds have a high incidence of retained deciduous teeth, which causes malpositioning of permanent teeth. Many lines of sheltie, for instance, have upper canines that jut straight forward because the roots of the deciduous teeth did not dissolve to allow the permanent to take their place.

A look at a moderate- or wild-type skull shows us what normal canine dentition should look like and how it should function (Figs. 11-1 and 11-2). The incisors are arranged in an arch (straighter on the bottom teeth) in which the crowns are aligned and touching, or nearly touching, edge to edge. The upper incisors lap over the lowers, and both occlude in a "scissors" arrangement (called a scissors bite) in which the crowns of one jaw pass so near those of the other as to shear food between them, like the blades of scissors. The function of the incisors is to provide delicate chewing action, such as picking shreds of

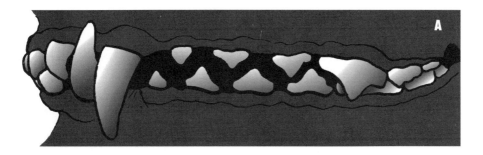

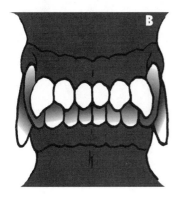

Figure 11-2

An illustration of a dog that has a good bite.
(A) Lateral view.
(B) Rostral view.

meat off of the bone or scratching an itch in the coat (grooming). They can also be used for holding or carrying things but do not stand up to severe pulling action because they can be exfoliated (pulled out) or broken too easily.

The canine teeth (a.k.a. fangs) have long, slightly curved roots that are about twice the length of those of incisors. The canines are intended to capture, puncture, and hold prey. They are the longest and most massive teeth in the dog's jaws. Because of the dog's instinct to use these teeth as tools, they are subject to excessive wear and/or fracture, as in "fence fighting," in which the dog chews or pulls at wire fencing.

The premolars, which generally have crowns that look like flattened triangles, function mainly as meat-cutting teeth. The natural arrangement of premolars calls for the crown of a tooth in one jaw to point between the premolars in the opposite jaw. The effect should be like interdigitating saw blades. The premolars do not touch each other but provide cutting, undulating surfaces to hold and process flesh.

The carnassial teeth—the upper fourth premolar and the lower first molar—are particularly useful for cutting flesh. In fact, the Latin prefix *carn-* means "flesh." The Latin root for meat, *carne*, is found in *chili con carne* ("chili with

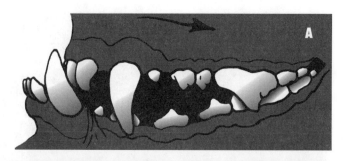
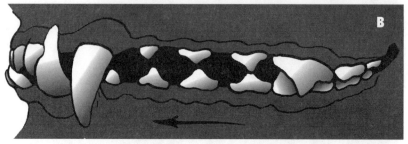
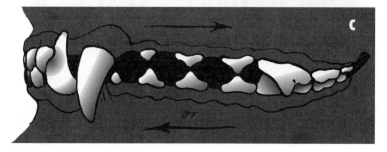

Figure 11-3

Examples of a type III malocclusion, with the lower jaw jutting out beyond the upper jaw: a brachycephalic bite (A), a prognathic bite (B), and an incipient type III malocclusion (C). In C, there is a level bite of the incisors, rather than the upper incisors lapping over the lower. The lower canine is thrust forward against the upper third incisor, and there is a gap between it and the upper canine. The premolars lack the normal zigzag orientation; since the lower premolars are half a tooth rostral of their normal position, crowns of the premolars point toward each other. This could be caused by a breeding program that emphasized a short face. Two dogs with this tendency would tend to produce offspring in which the lower incisors are rostral to the upper, a malocclusion that is a fault in any breed other than the brachycephalics.

meat"). Unlike the other premolars, the carnassials are situated one above the other, and they work by overlapping in a scissors action, with the upper tooth passing just lateral to and almost in contact with the lower. The long cutting edges of the crowns of these teeth are narrow and sharp, and they cut meat (or your best shoes) into digestible chunks.

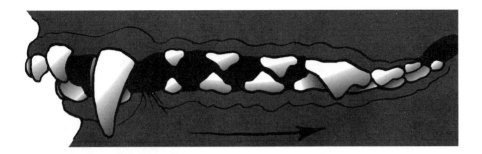

Figure 11-4
Type II malocclusion. Here the lower jaw is exceptionally short.

The most caudal portion of the lower first molar is low, flat, and blunt, and it interdigitates with the upper first molar in the dog. Molars (two on the top, and three on the bottom) are generally flat, low-crowned teeth that are useful for grinding coarse food of vegetable origin. They are the best evidence that the dog is truly an omnivore, an animal that can chew up and digest food other than meat. The cat has only pointed, carnivore teeth (including the molars).

Most malocclusions have to do with the growth and development of the bones of the jaws rather than the placement of the teeth within the bones. In fact, there are three general categories of malocclusions. Type III has already been discussed; it occurs because the face is relatively shorter than the lower jaw. It is commonly called an underbite or an underslung or undershot jaw. A brachycephalic dog has a normal-length mandible, but the face is foreshortened (Fig. 11-3A). Less frequent are prognathic mandibles, which are longer than normal (Fig. 11-3B). To determine whether the face is short or the mandible long, compare the lengths to those of an average dog of the same size.

Type II is the opposite situation, where the upper jaw is relatively long as compared with the lower. In Figure 11-4, the lower canine cannot erupt between the upper third incisor and upper canine and is consequently perforating the palate medial to the upper canine. Such a bite is very painful during eruption and should be corrected in the puppy by extracting the lower canines and in the young adult by crown reduction and pulp capping (also called vital pulpotomy). See Chapter 10 for this procedure.

Type I is a condition where the jaws are relatively normal, but individual teeth are misplaced in the arcade (Fig. 11-5). One example is the lance tooth, where a retained deciduous upper canine causes rostral deflection of the permanent upper canine (Fig. 11-6A). This will result in interference with the lower

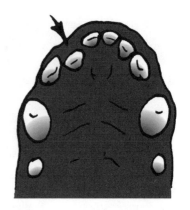

Figure 11-5

Type I malocclusion. Although the arches of the jaws and their orientation to each other are normal, this animal shows a tooth that is out of place in the upper arcade (*arrow*). A tooth in the wrong place may be caused by a misplaced tooth bud or a retained deciduous tooth.

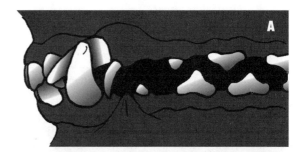

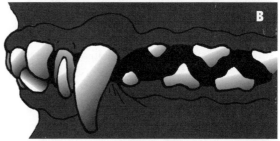

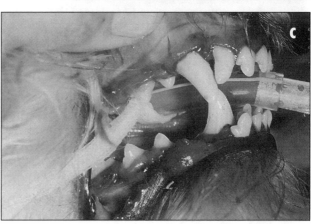

Figure 11-6

The lance tooth (A) and base-narrow canine (B) are type I malocclusions. (C) This unfortunate dog has both a lance tooth and a base-narrow canine due to retained deciduous teeth, which are no longer present but were there as the permanent teeth were erupting.

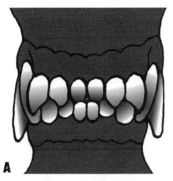

Figure 11-7

(A) Dropped incisors, a type I malocclusion.

(B) This dog has an exaggerated version of dropped incisors. The original crowding of the incisors occurred because of base-narrow canines (note how the canines are directly behind the third incisors instead of slightly lateral and caudal).

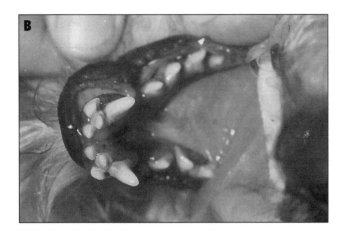

canine, which completes the malpositioning of the upper canine. This condition is common in certain breeds or lines of dog, most notably in the Shetland sheepdog. Another deviation is the base-narrow canine (Fig. 11-6B): medial deviation of the lower permanent canines results from retained deciduous lower canines, and the permanent teeth often perforate the palate.

Other common type I malocclusions are dropped incisors and the anterior cross-bite. Dropped incisors often occur because of crowding in the lower jaw (Fig. 11-7). The first (middle) mandibular incisors are thrust forward and are not in place behind the upper first incisors. The second incisors are commonly stepped back out of the arch, and the third incisors are forward in a more normal position caudal to the upper incisors. In the anterior cross-bite, the lower right second and third incisors are in front of the upper incisors (Fig. 11-8).

The wry bite is in a classification of its own because one side of the face (both upper and lower jaws) grows more than the other. In the wry bite, the midline of the teeth does not line up, and one side of the mouth has an "open" bite—

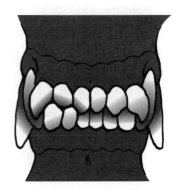

Figure 11-8

Anterior cross-bite, a type I malocclusion. Notice how the lower right (to the left in the drawing) second and third incisors are in front of the upper incisors. This could have been caused by retained upper deciduous second and third incisors.

there are larger spaces between the teeth (see the open bite in Fig. 11-9). Dogs with a wry bite usually show asymmetry of the skull as well, unless the asymmetry seen in the teeth has been caused by localized trauma to the smaller side of the head. Unless bone growth has been caused by trauma, it is considered very heritable, and such dogs should not be bred. A wry bite may be severe or very subtle, which is mainly evident on an X ray. In many cases it can be treated like a type I malocclusion.

The simplest type of malocclusion to change is type I. Because the jaws themselves are in misalignment, types II and III can only be re-aligned to occlude more correctly if the malocclusions are rather mild.

Any time teeth strike other teeth or soft tissue, there is a potential for pain; this is a viable reason for orthodontic therapy in dogs. Unfortunately, dog owners and handlers have used orthodontics not as a therapeutic option but strictly for cosmetics. If two dogs are essentially the same, but one has a crooked tooth, it doesn't take a rocket scientist to figure out that the dog with the straight teeth will win in a dog show. In the throes of unhealthy competition, owners will resort to surgery or orthodontics to get the edge over the competition. Neither alteration of a dog's appearance is allowed under present Kennel Club rules. The reason why is obvious—every physical trait, unless it has been caused by some sort of environmental influence—is heritable. The American Kennel Club utilizes shows to promote the "best" individuals of a breed so that these animals will be pursued for breeding. If they have been cosmetically altered, they will still, of course, pass on "undesirable" traits to their offspring.

Dog show people pursue veterinarians who perform orthodontics on dogs. Many veterinarians, to avoid being complicit in a fraudulent action, provide a statement that clients must sign that declares that they will not show the dog or will neuter it (neutered animals are not allowed in breed classes). The determined competitor will sign the statement knowing full well that he or

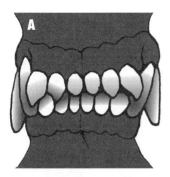

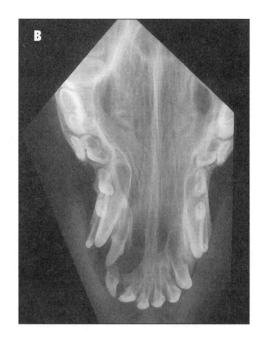

Figure 11-9

Wry bite, a type I malocclusion.

(A) Notice that the midline of the teeth does not line up, and the left side of the mouth (to the right in the drawing) has an "open" bite.

(B) Note the lack of symmetry in the dog's maxillary X ray.

she intends to campaign the dog. Although few people will spend the money involved in cosmetic orthodontic treatment for a pet, there are some who will do so simply for aesthetics. It should be remembered, however, that if a dog is a purebred, it is a representative of its breeding line and can be used as an example by breeders even if neutered. It is very important that orthodontics clients be screened for intent; nobody likes to be used for deceitful purposes.

Orthodontics performed to prevent or alleviate pain generally falls in a separate category than those procedures done purely for cosmetics. Many of the animals that need correction (as for base-narrow canines, for instance) come from pet stocks or are nonpurebreds. The service provided for these animals can mean the difference between misery and a pain-free existence. No animal is entitled to a perfect bite, but as stewards of our pets, we are obliged to give them a comfortable existence.

Orthodontics for the Base-Narrow Canine

The base-narrow lower canine is the most common malocclusion. One or both of the mandibular canines may be base-narrow. When the root of the lower deciduous canine does not regress in response to the development of the permanent tooth, it will prevent the permanent tooth from assuming the normal position in the mouth. The permanent lower tooth will erupt medially (inside the mouth) relative to the deciduous. A dog's lower jaw is notice-

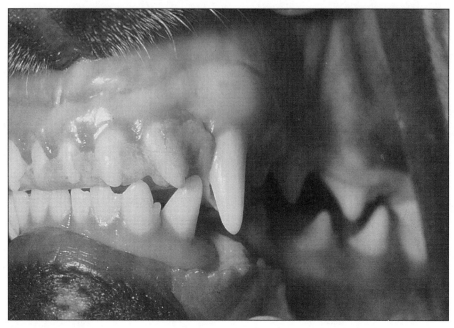

Figure 11-10

Appearance of the acrylic inclined plane for base-narrow canines in a dog's mouth. The acrylic, which is visible between the incisors and in front of the upper canine tooth, protects the palate and deflects the lower canines laterally.

ably narrower than the upper jaw, and in order for the lower canines to avoid striking the palate, they must flare dramatically laterally. If a canine is prevented from flaring laterally by a deciduous canine still in place, it will erupt straight up. Every time the dog closes its mouth, it will traumatize the soft tissue (and eventually the bone) of the palate—fistulas from mouth into nose have been created by canine teeth. This trauma is painful. And even if the retained deciduous tooth is removed, the permanent tooth will not shift into place because the hole created in the palatal mucosa acts like an elastic retainer every time the dog closes its mouth.

If the permanent canine is striking the palate just medial to its proper position, and there is adequate space for it to rest between the upper third incisor and the canine, the orthodontic treatment can be relatively fast and easy. If it is still present, the deciduous canine must be extracted. Then an acrylic appliance is formed on the upper arcade (Fig. 11-10) after etching the teeth to make the acrylic stick to them. The acrylic that covers the palate has a ramp formed into it so that when the tooth strikes it is deflected into the proper position. The acrylic inclined plane may be used for unilateral or bilateral base-narrow canines, but it is important that if there is only one to be corrected that the other have a formed area in the acrylic as well, or the jaw could merely twist to the affected side.

In a young dog, the jaws are still growing—and base-narrow canines should be corrected in as young a dog as possible. Since part of the growth is the widening of the maxilla, the upper canines should not be encased in acrylic; the appliance should simply be abutted to their inside edges, with the adhesion to the incisors being the main retention for the appliance. In the older dog, the upper canines may be surrounded by the acrylic to more effectively anchor the device.

As the technician, you can help with the anesthetizing of the animal by cleaning any calculus off the teeth before beginning and by positioning the animal dorsally so that the palate is easy to work on.

The next step is to acid etch the teeth intended to anchor the device. The acid comes in a gel or solution, which is applied by syringe or disposable dental brush, respectively. The exposure time differs by product, and you can keep the time and have the air/water syringe ready. The acid is thoroughly rinsed off of teeth and soft tissues (a gauze sponge can be used to catch the gel or the majority of the dissolved liquid acid before it spreads excessively). Then the teeth are dried, and a tooth surface that does not appear chalky (dull) is re-etched.

Acrylic may be applied as powder followed by liquid chemical with a dam around the teeth to keep it from running off (the dam can be made of window caulk or other soft, malleable material). However, this technique is slow and tedious, and I prefer to mix the approximate amount needed for the entire device at one time. Do not use plastic or wax-coated containers for mixing because these will tend to melt. Plain paper cups are too porous. I use discarded, clean glass jars (baby-food-size are best) or empty, clean cans with a tongue depressor or wooden handle of a cotton applicator to mix the material.

Mixing the acrylic may be assigned to you. The approximate amount of powder is poured into the container (generally 3–4 cc), and the liquid is added until the powder is just wetted. Then the mixture is stirred until it becomes sticky and begins to wad up. The wad can be formed by hand, especially if your hands have been lightly covered with petrolatum. The acrylic is pressed onto the incisor teeth, it is molded to the approximate shape of the ramp for the teeth, and the mouth is closed (this may require removing the endotracheal tube or simply taking it loose and doubling it briefly into the animal's mouth or pushing it farther down the throat to allow the teeth to find their natural position). Then the veterinary dentist can take the soft acrylic out to set, being careful not to distort the impression of the teeth, or it can be left in place. Dental acrylic is very exothermic (it releases heat) as it solidifies. Cold water run over and under it as it heats will decrease the amount of burn to

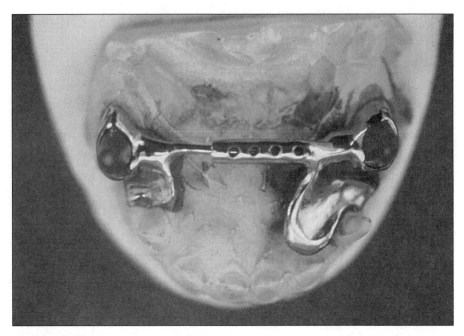

Figure 11-11

Telescoping inclined plane for a base-narrow canine on a stone model of a dog's upper jaw. The anchors are the canine teeth, and metal wings flare in front of the canines to capture the tips of the lower canines. Note that the right wing (*on the right side of the photo*) is longer and extends medially over the palate. The right lower canine is the one that is base-narrow. A wing must also be made for the normal (*left*) lower canine because the lower jaw would tend to twist if only one lower canine was caught by the appliance.

Photo courtesy of Dr. Ed Eisner.

the palate, which can otherwise be severe. The thicker the acrylic, the hotter the material gets, and thermal damage can be injurious to the teeth as well as to soft tissues.

If the appliance is cured outside the mouth, it needs to be cemented in place with more acrylic, and alternating powder and liquid chemical are used to do this. Whether the appliance cures in or out of the mouth, to reform the ramp, the gap in the acrylic left by the misplaced tooth is filled the same way. Prior to inserting the appliance, the appliance and mouth must be dry before applying the acrylic powder and liquid.

A dog generally wakes up fighting the appliance in its mouth but seldom can displace it. Surprisingly, the teeth usually move to the correct position in about two weeks because every time the dog closes its mouth it is applying pressure to move the tooth. If the mouth can close entirely but the correction is inadequate, a thicker acrylic layer is applied to the ramp during a second anesthesia. It is desirable to get a millimeter or two overcorrection because the periodontal fibers of the recently moved tooth tend to make it rebound a bit. However, once the dentist is satisfied with the movement, the appliance may be removed.

By the end of a two-week period, the acrylic will become brittle, and saliva will have recalcified the enamel of the teeth that were acid etched so the acrylic will lose adhesion. There will still be some mechanical retention, however, and the acrylic generally must be cracked off the teeth with extraction forceps until the entire appliance can be pulled off. Most dogs tolerate this awake, but some may need to be briefly anesthetized.

Clients must be informed that the appliance will retain food material and sloughing mucosa and so will tend to become odoriferous. The client can minimize the odor by rinsing the mouth with a syringe containing an oral disinfectant, such as 1–2 percent chlorhexidine. The gingiva invariably becomes inflamed; happily, this resolves once the appliance is removed.

The palate itself will act as a retainer for the tooth because the dog usually spends a good part of its day with its mouth closed, so the tooth cannot return to its former maloccluded position.

Conventional Orthodontics for Other Malocclusions

The big advantage to the acrylic inclined plane for base-narrow canines is that it is a type of "one-stop shopping," which most clients prefer. However, other malocclusions must be handled in a more traditional way: dental models and an impression are made, the appliance is produced in a laboratory, the appliance is fitted, and the appliance is constantly monitored and adjusted once it is in place. Base-narrow canines can be treated in this way, too (Fig. 11-11).

The first step in orthodontics is to make a mold of the dog's mouth as it looks on presentation. In human dentistry, the technician often does this, and you may be trained to do it as well. Of course, the dog must be anesthetized (people who have suffered full-mouth impressions probably wish they could have been anesthetized instead of suffering the gagging sensation of having the wet mold material shoved deep into their mouths). The mold material is called alginate. It comes in a powder that is mixed with water to make a thick, gel-like substance that resembles thickened wheat paste. Some veterinary dentists like to mix their own alginate, but many prefer an assistant to do so.

The alginate comes with instructions regarding proportions of powder to water, but ambient humidity or aridity can throw off these ratios. Most people who mix alginate add a thin dribble of water until the alginate reaches the right consistency. The alginate must be mixed rapidly and used quickly. It is mixed in a rubber mixing bowl with a plastic spatula. The bowl is held in the palm of one hand while the spatula is rapidly beaten against the side and bottom. Once the consistency is right—it holds itself up without sagging yet is soft enough to easily make an impression in it, and it is wet on the surface—the stuff is pressed into a mold form, and care is taken not to create any air pockets.

Manufactured mold forms (trays) come in several sizes. They have holes all over the surface for the alginate to ooze out of as the impression is made. Prior to making the mold, you, the technician, should check the trays against the dog's jaw to make sure that they are long enough and wide enough—at least 6 mm, or 1/4 in., outside the edges of the jaw to give a good impression. The dog is placed on its sternum or back with whatever jaw is the target being "up" so that the tray need not be held upside down—alginate may be lost. The alginate is pressed up on the teeth until they disappear. It is best to include several millimeters of gingiva so that the finished model will be at least 12 mm, or ½ in., thick. The tray is then held firmly in place without moving for a few minutes until the alginate is set. If you aren't certain how firm it can get, it is better to give it a little more time because when it first sets it is more fragile. However, once really firm, the alginate is rubbery, and the slight rocking action to remove the tray will not mar it.

The set alginate is only a temporary mold. It generally has a useful shelf life of 45 minutes or less, because it will naturally begin to desiccate (dry) in the air. If the model is not to be poured immediately, the alginate should be protected from drying by enclosing in a plastic bag with wet paper towels. Drying causes shrinking of the alginate, distorting the tooth impressions.

The next step is the pouring of the mold. Dental stone (a material like plaster of paris) comes as a powder and, like alginate, must be mixed into a liquid to be used. A model vibrator should be set up before mixing the stone; it should be covered with plastic to keep the liquid material from coating it. The very first stone that is mixed (in the same manner as alginate) should be runny, like a milk shake. Only a small quantity is made this consistency, just to fill the tips of the teeth. The stone tries to make air bubbles, even when this thin, and it should be forced gently down to the tips of the tooth impressions. The wooden handle of a cotton applicator can be used to carefully push the air bubbles out, and the vibrator finishes the job. Once the bubbles stop appearing from the vibrations, the mixture for the next layer of stone may be made and poured. This layer needs to be poured immediately, or there will be no bond between the first and second layers. It can be thicker than the first, as it does not have to flow into tooth tips; it forms the tooth shapes and gingival margins. It, too, is vibrated to remove any little bubbles. Finally, to thicken the stone model for strength, a last layer of stone is added before the second

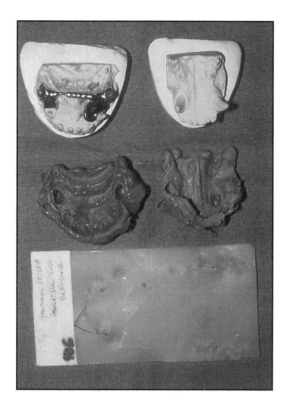

Figure 11-12

Cast stone models, top, with manufactured appliance in place. The objects in the middle are rubber impressions, and the one on the bottom is a wax bite registration.

Photo courtesy of Dr. Ed Eisner.

one is set. This can be mixed quite thick and layered and formed with the spatula to a certain extent. It can even be cut to a pleasing tapered block shape instead of being ground down with a model trimmer. Then the stone is allowed to set for 1–2 hours.

Before the dog is awakened, a flat piece of impression wax (Fig. 11-12) large enough to lay between the teeth of the opposing jaws is heated in hot water (in a large bowl, usually) and taken out when it is malleable. The dog is extubated, and the jaws clamped closed over the wax until it cools and firms up (almost immediately). This will give the lab an exact impression of how the crowns of the teeth come together. Another help for the lab is to use a fine-tipped marker to draw a line from the tip of the canine tooth across to the opposite gingiva on the model once it is finished, using the position of the real dog's teeth as a visual guide to how the teeth fit together (Fig. 11-13). This is strictly an "eyeball" exercise, and if one is not good at estimating proportions, it should not be done.

Cleanup of alginate and stone is a challenge; it is usually the technician's job and is always a messy proposition. The majority of the alginate and stone on equipment should be cleaned over the wastebasket. Both alginate and stone

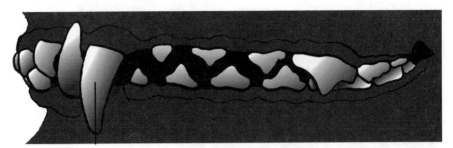

Figure 11-13

A line can be drawn on the model that shows where the canine teeth strike.

can clog plumbing. It is best to have a plaster trap if using stone, but if a trap is not available, nothing should be washed down the sink but tiny quantities of stone with lots of water—like washing off root vegetables from the garden (the majority of the dirt is removed before they are brought into the house). The sink should have a strainer in the drain to catch any small pieces of alginate or stone. Both materials scrape and peel off of the rubber bowl readily once they have set. Paper towels can be used to wipe out still-liquid materials. Dispose of paper towels in the wastebasket.

The stone model must be removed from the alginate while the latter is still rubbery (while stone generally needs 12 hours to set well, alginate will stay rubbery for several hours). A knife should first be run around the inside of the tray to allow the alginate to loosen from its sides. Any alginate that has flowed through the bottom holes in the tray should be trimmed off as well. The alginate and stone imbedded in it can then be pulled out of the tray. The teeth in the model are much more fragile than the real things, and just trying to peel the alginate off will fracture stone tooth crowns. Therefore, the alginate should be cut and peeled in sections, with special care taken over the canines. If a tooth tip does break off, it can be repaired with white glue, but it is critical that it is in exact alignment. If there is a slight gap from an air bubble in the stone, it may be carefully patched with some more stone. If there is a bulge on the tooth or gingiva, there was a bubble in the alginate. These can be carved off with a sharp knife. It is important that these repairs not be done on a critical tooth—say, one that is to have a crown prep (see below) or one that is scheduled to carry a fitted appliance.

The final finish of a stone model is intended to grind off rough edges and, if desired, to even out the sides, top, and bottom. This is done with a model trimmer carrying a large, Carborundum wheel bathed in water. This machine should never be emptied into a drain without a plaster trap. It can be drained into a container or onto the ground, if used outside, but the amount of stone ground off during a finish of a model is almost guaranteed to stop up a conventional drain.

Models are sent to laboratories with specific instructions about what needs to be done and what type of appliance the veterinary dentist desires. The majority of appliances are of cast metal, but some may have components of other materials, especially acrylic. Sometimes the veterinarian will ask the advice of the lab about how to approach a certain problem. The challenges inherent in orthodonture for dogs, although similar to those of people, are different in several ways. The patient's compliance, for instance, may differ. Appliances for dogs generally must be tougher than those for people, and labs for human dentistry may not be able to make adequate appliances for dogs. There are a very small number of labs in the United States prepared to make canine appliances, and the model must be shipped to them. The model must be protected from breakage in shipping (usually this involves wrapping individual halves separately in bubble wrap and surrounding everything with styrofoam "popcorn").

When the appliance returns, it is fitted on the model to make certain it will go onto the teeth properly to do its job. Then you anesthetize the dog and position it for the easiest placement of the particular appliance onto the teeth. The teeth to which the appliance will attach are treated according to the instructions for the cement to be used. The surface of the appliance that is attached to the tooth may be roughened; sandblasting is a favorite technique (miniature sandblasters are available for this purpose). After cleaning and roughening the surface, it should not be touched without gloves because skin oils can prevent adhesion. A variety of adhesives are used to attach appliances; they should be strong enough to last for months but ideally not be difficult to remove (this is a hard combination to achieve). The technician can prove useful here by mixing and having cement ready when the appliance is ready to go on. Typically, the appliance is set and held in place for several minutes to assure a good bond, depending upon the adhesive.

Frequent rechecks are a necessity with orthodonture; if rechecks are included in the price of the appliance, people will be more likely to keep their appointments (although this is not necessarily so). Educating the client about the importance of rechecks and following directions on adjustments is critical. The clients often do the adjustments. Adjustments usually involve inserting a hex key into a socket and twisting a quarter of a turn (Fig. 11-14). Orthodonture must proceed slowly, by tiny increments, with long-term, light, steady pressure. The purpose is to push the teeth through the bone (which will remodel to accommodate the movement) while retaining the viability of the periodontal ligament. If there is too much pressure applied, the cells of the periodontal ligament will be squashed and killed; this will lead to fusion to bone and eventual resorption of the root. Besides this, too much pressure is painful to the patient.

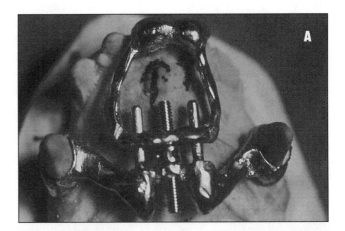

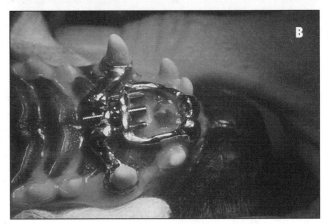

Figure 11-14

(A) An appliance fitted to a model of the rostral upper jaw. The appliance is designed to correct the anterior cross-bite.

(B) The appliance in place on the dog. A screw mechanism will be turned on a regular basis to push the affected teeth forward. A key fits into the appliance to turn it. Most dogs tolerate this very well.

Photos courtesy of Dr. Ed Eisner.

The type of orthodonture that requires an appliance is often one in which a pushing pressure away from a tooth or teeth is utilized. When traction can be used, an appliance may not be necessary. The main thing to remember is that the tooth that is the anchor (whether to push or to pull) must be more strongly rooted than the one that must be moved. Because big teeth, like the canines, are likely to be out of place, binding more than one tooth together to pull them may be required. A lance tooth, a condition in which the upper canine is prevented from erupting into place just behind the lower canine because of a retained deciduous tooth and instead shoots straight forward, is an example of this (Fig. 11-15). The upper canine is fastened via an elastic to the upper fourth premolar, which in turn is solidly connected to the first molar behind it.

Brackets are attached to the teeth involved by use of a cement, as are lab-constructed appliances. These brackets have spools, loops, or hooks on which to fasten wires and elastic chain or rubber bands. The elastic chain (called a Masel chain) is first applied with almost no tension; the chain is shortened on

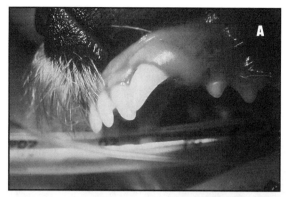

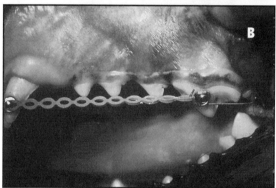

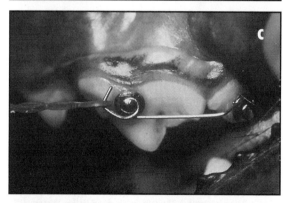

Figure 11-15

(A) Lance tooth due to retained deciduous teeth.

(B) Brackets are cemented to teeth (canine, upper fourth premolar, and first molar), and a Masel chain attached.

(C) Appearance of the brackets on the rear teeth. These teeth are wired together to give a more substantial anchor to move the massively rooted canine.

(D) Appearance of the canine tooth near the time of removal of the brackets and chain. It is now in the correct position.

Photos courtesy of Dr. Ed Eisner.

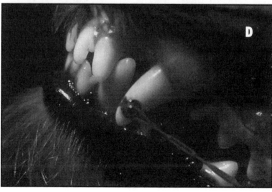

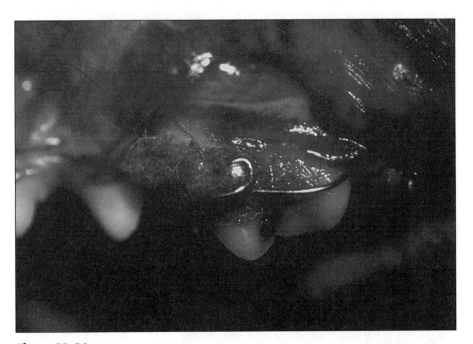

Figure 11-16

Hygiene is very important when orthodontic devices are used. Notice the accumulation of plaque and debris on the brackets of the case. This can predispose the animal to periodontitis and will create an obnoxious odor.

Photo courtesy of Dr. Ed Eisner.

a schedule until the tooth is in place. Owners can count links of the Masel chain and progressively tighten them to order. Owners also can change elastic bands or Masel chains if they should break or lose elasticity.

The removal of brackets or cemented appliances requires anesthesia. Occasionally a spring-loaded crown remover or cushioned forceps can be utilized to pop an appliance or a bracket off the teeth, but occasionally it must be cut off the anchoring teeth. This must be done very carefully (usually with diamond burs to cut metal) to avoid damaging the enamel. The cement often can be lifted off the tooth with an ultrasonic scaler, but if not, it also must be carefully cleaned off the tooth with finishing burs, stones, and/or abrasive discs. A thorough cleaning of the teeth is indicated after appliance removal.

Appliances are usually left in place for a long time (often several months) because of the tendency for a tooth to shift back toward its former position, so home care is very important. The teeth must be brushed thoroughly around the appliance or brackets every day because they accumulate foodstuff and plaque and have no chance of self-cleaning (Fig. 11-16). In addition, the toys and chew aids that the dog might ordinarily chew on are forbidden during orthodonture because they can break or dislodge expensive appliances. It would be a shame if expensive orthodontic procedures were useless because of teeth lost to periodontitis.

PROSTHODONTICS

In human dentistry, we are accustomed to seeing or hearing about full or partial sets of false teeth, individual false teeth, crowns, onlays ("caps"), and bridges. In cats, because of the size of the teeth, prosthodontics are impractical except for canines. Prosthodontics are not common in the dog world either, although any of the above can be performed on dogs. The limiting factors are expense and the excessive force dogs often apply to teeth. The most often seen prosthodontic in veterinary dentistry is a full crown (Figs. 11-17 and 11-18).

The crown, a snug-fitting casing, provides some protection for the remaining tooth beneath. In order to apply the crown, the tooth must be reduced in size to allow the crown to fit with the other teeth; this removal of enamel and dentin potentially weakens the tooth.

There are several indications for a crown. One is a tooth that has been subject to excessive wear, as in fence-fighting, and is in danger of a pathological fracture or pulp exposure. Another is a devitalized tooth, such as an upper fourth premolar that has died and become brittle; this tooth, particularly if it has suffered a slab fracture open to the pulp due to unhealthy chewing habits, is in danger of additional fracture after root canal therapy. (The upper fourth premolar, the carnassial tooth, is subject to a slab being cracked off the outside when narrow hard objects are chewed.) The two most common teeth to receive full crowns are the two that suffer the most trauma and breakage: the upper fourth premolars and the canines. Crowns can be cast in several metals (titanium, gold, etc.), or may have porcelain bonded to metal on one or more sides, or may be made of special fibered ceramics—essentially the same choices that a human recipient might have. Metal crowns are usually used for dogs.

One of the limitations of using crowns in dogs is the tremendous stress they receive when the dog bites down. Law enforcement service dogs use their teeth to bite, apprehend, and hold suspects; they must be trained to do this properly and constantly drilled to maintain their edge. These dogs are often very enthusiastic about their work and will attack a metal door as readily as a suspect if it is asked of them, or they will go through barriers to apprehend someone. Unfortunately this puts their teeth at risk for breakage or excessive wear (abrasion). Police dogs have been retired because their teeth are no longer adequate for their job. Although dogs are trained to bite with their

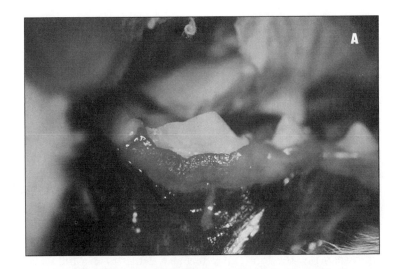

Figure 11-17

(A) Left upper fourth premolar (this dog is on its back) that has been fractured and given a root canal. To prepare this tooth for a crown that will protect it from further fracture, the enamel and some dentin is ground off the width of the crown. Then a model of both jaws is cast, showing how much space the lab must leave when making the crown.

(B) The crown on a portion of the stone model.

(C) The metal crown cemented in place.

Photos courtesy of Dr. Ed Eisner.

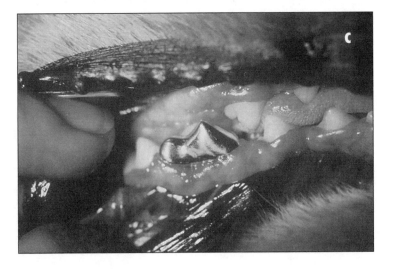

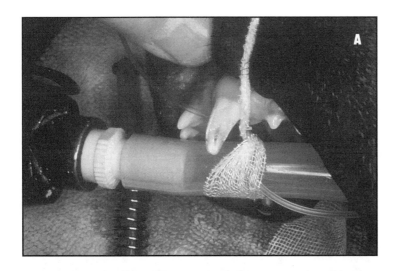

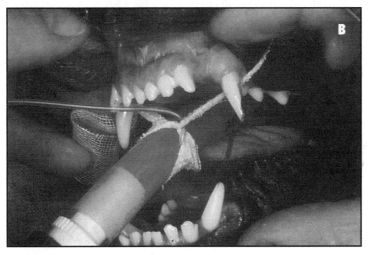

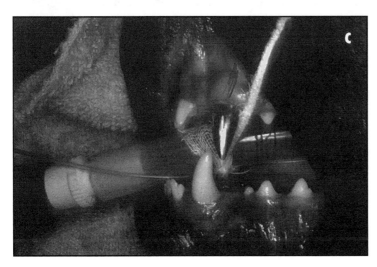

Figure 11-18

(A) A fractured canine that will need endodontal treatment prior to preparation for the crown.

(B) The tooth ground down and ready for the impression tray.

(C) The finished metal crown. Crowns are also available in porcelain bonded to metal.

Photos courtesy of Dr. Ed Eisner.

entire mouths, the most wear usually occurs in the front teeth. The force that large police dogs can exert with their jaws is phenomenal. Attempts have been made to quantify the force, with equivocal success. Estimates of 1000 psi (pounds per square inch) have been made. Then there is the shearing force on the teeth. The natural instinct of a dog in a fighting mode is to pull and shake quarry, which puts lateral and rostral stress on the teeth.

The shearing forces are the ones that usually cause problems for canine crowns. The obvious hope of the police department with a dog with worn or broken canines is to restore them to their full length. However, if there is no dentin to support the tips of the crowns, there is increased shearing force at the base of the crown, and the entire crown will kink and/or come off, or the tooth will break off at the crown/root interface. Realistically, to prevent this from happening, crowns cannot be more than 2–3 mm longer than the existing tooth.

The first step in crown preparation is to carve down the crown of the tooth to prepare it for the permanent prosthodontic. If the tooth has an elaborate shape, like some upper fourth premolars, it must be remodeled so it has a gradual taper, because the crown will not go onto a tooth that is thinner at the gum line than at the distal portion. If there is a very tight fit with an adjacent tooth (as in the canine tooth interlock), particular care must be taken to grind off adequate enamel and dentin for the thickness of the crown (usually 1.5-2 mm). Then the margin of the crown prep must be made. Although there are several ways to make the crown interdigitate with the dentin of the tooth, the most successful is probably with a camber. The cambered edge of the tooth is about one-fourth of a circle so that the crown edge is not too thin and yet does not end abruptly, which would be more difficult to cement properly. The crown prep is usually performed with round and tapered burs.

Once the crown prep is complete (this is always done after any endodontic therapy), a full-mouth stone model is made, as for orthodontic appliances. In addition, because the detail of the crown prep usually is not perfect with a stone model, an impression is made of the tooth with rubber-based material; this impression will be sent with the stone model to the lab for confirmation of the shape of the crown prep.

Usually, in human dentistry we are sent home with temporary crowns—plastic shapes that will protect the peglike crown prep. Since dogs have such varying shapes and sizes of teeth, there are no generic shapes for temporary crowns, as there are for humans. Until the dog returns for the crown, the owner must take care that the dog has no opportunity to fracture the unprotected prepped tooth because any deficit will affect the retention of the crown.

As soon as the lab returns the model and the crown, the crown is checked to make sure it fits the model and then, after the dog is anesthetized, the tooth. The tooth and crown are cleaned and dried; care must be taken not to touch the surfaces to be cemented. It is critical that the interior surface of the crown be roughened, and if the lab has not sandblasted it, this must be done at the hospital. There are several cements (called luting cements) that are useful for attaching crowns. One thing that several have in common is that once mixed they do not set up as long as they are exposed to oxygen. The technician usually has the task of constantly moving the cement with a spatula by pressing it flat and scraping it up to keep it exposed to the air. When the crown is ready for the final application, its inside and the tooth are coated with cement. The crown is then applied and held in place for a few minutes (depending on the type of cement), after which any excess cement is cleaned off from the margins. Margins should be as smooth as possible because irregularities create pockets for plaque to form.

Most crown margins are made supragingivally (coronally from the gum line). Subgingival margins tend to create small voids between tooth and crown. These lead to gingivitis or periodontitis, which, in turn, usually results in gingival recession over time unless painstaking home care is practiced.

When a tooth is broken off near the gum line, a client may want the tooth for aesthetic reasons. After endodontic therapy is performed, a plastic post is imbedded into the root with restorative. The stone model and impression are made of the post sticking out of the tooth; then the post is removed, and the gingiva sutured over the root until the crown is ready. The crown comes back with a metal post embedded in it; this is the crown and post technique. When it is cemented, the crown and post is prepared similarly to a regular crown. This type of crown is very susceptible to damage.

Another rather fragile technique for a lost tooth, if the root is missing, is to create a false tooth (called a pontic) and to attach it to two or more adjacent teeth with a bridge. This technique is fairly common in human dentistry, where the recipients can guard against breaking the bridge, which is usually a laboratory-constructed appliance from a stone model. The false tooth is not functional: it floats in space just above the gingiva and is obviously only added for aesthetic reasons.

RESTORATIVE DENTISTRY

We are most familiar with dental restoratives as the "fillings" that have been placed in our teeth to repair caries. Restoratives are also used to seal the entrance holes for endodontal procedures and to repair minor chips or deficits in the tooth surface. The most important thing to remember with restoratives is that there is nothing that can be put into a tooth that will make that tooth as strong as it was before the restoration.

Amalgam Restorations

There are generally three types of restorations placed in the mouth. The most common has been amalgam because it is the strongest material found that can replace the normal tooth enamel and dentin. Amalgam is mostly a mixture of the liquid metal mercury and silver powder. It becomes a silvery gray metallic or darker color in the mouth. For a short time after it has been mixed, it is somewhat malleable, although crumbly. It is packed into the tooth with metal instruments (condensers) by layers until it has completely filled the deficit, then carved to the exact level, then burnished and polished smooth.

The technician is almost always responsible for the mixing of restoratives. Fortunately, since mercury is so poisonous, amalgam is no longer mixed by hand but is available in premeasured ampules shaped like tiny plastic barrels. These are placed in a special agitating machine with two little arms that hold the ampule. The machine, called an amalgamator, can also be used to mix certain premeasured nonmetal restoratives packaged in similar ampules. The product information indicates the time required for mixing. The amalgam is not mixed until the tooth prep is completed. This may involve applying an intermediate restorative material (see below) prior to the amalgam.

To have good access to the amalgam, it is placed in a small but thick glass container called a dappen dish. Amalgam is transported into the tooth by use of an amalgam carrier. This instrument is useful for other materials as well and is always used in the same way. The powdery, crumbly, or semisolid material is collected in the tube of the carrier by pressing the tube in the material until it is full. Then the tube is placed over the tooth, and a trigger squeezed that pushes a plunger through the tube, emptying it. Amalgam carriers come in several diameters to accommodate different sizes of cavities into which the malleable metal is placed. Once the amalgam begins to harden, it will no longer be workable with a condenser or burnisher, and more will have to be made if the cavity prep is not filled.

Amalgam has lost favor with veterinary and human dentists, who have gone largely to the composites and glass ionomers. Disadvantages of the amalgam include appearance, health considerations, and requirements for mechanical retention. In most mouths, the silvery surface of the amalgam turns more dark gray, and amalgam tends to stain dentin gray (turning a tooth dark), especially if a restoration is extensive. In humans, amalgam restorations have been shown to leach metallic mercury, which, as mentioned above, can be quite poisonous. Mercury can cause a variety of health problems, but it is especially toxic to the developing nervous system. Its effects are cumulative, and it stays in the body for years. All restorations benefit from mechanical retention (a slight undercut in the deepest portion of the restoration); of restoration materials only the glass ionomers and some composites adhere to dentin and can be used on the surface of dentin without mechanical retention as long as the restored teeth aren't subject to shearing forces.

Alternatives to Amalgam

The greatest advantage of the composites and glass ionomers is that they can be selected by color to match the teeth. Both have filling materials of silica, quartz, or other similar substances for strength in the base substance and may be found as chemically or light-cured products. They generally are available as a malleable, thick paste and then set up hard in the tooth. They were first available as a powder/liquid that could be mixed to a paste, and powdered products are still available. Both composites and glass ionomers have a tendency to "slump," similar to a thick liquidlike molasses, if layered too thick or if curing is delayed.

Curing of Alternatives

▶ Chemically Cured Restoratives

The chemical cures involve mixing a catalyst with the base resin. As in any chemical reaction, the time to cure depends on ambient temperature—the higher the temperature, the faster the chemical reaction that results in hardening of the restoration. Several things will adversely affect chemical curing of these restoratives. Water or oil may prevent hardening. Also, any substance on the wall of the preparation that prevents the restoration from fitting tight against the tooth will foster leakage. For instance, if dentin powder was left in place on the prepared wall, it could eventually erode and allow fluid to seep down the prepared surface.

▶ Light-Cured Restoratives

The light-cured restoratives involve using a curing light to make the preparation harden. The restoration often must be made in layers because light generally will not penetrate more than a couple of millimeters. The light-cured restoratives first produced (composites) were sensitive only to ultraviolet light. Unfortunately, UV light can be damaging to eyes, so it was dangerous to use, even when (human) patients wore special glasses. The curing lights now used cover the visible spectrum and are safer, although they are intense enough to cause eye damage if looked at directly (like looking at the sun). Even light reflected off the teeth can be too bright to look at directly. As anesthetized veterinary patients can't be told not to look into the light, the eyes of dogs and cats should be covered to avoid injury to them with curing lights.

The curing lights have filters to protect the user's eyes while aiming the lights at the animal's mouth. If you cannot look through the filter because it is angled for the person using the light, you should avert your eyes. Only one person, the one actually holding the light, needs to see that the light is still on target, and he or she can direct it while looking through the filter. Curing lights have preset times corresponding to the needs of the particular product. You should make sure that the time is set correctly because once the trigger is pulled the light will be on for the full preset time and keeping the light on longer than it needs to be uses up the life of the bulb. Since there can be inadvertent curing of a restoration by other bright lights, such as a powerful exam light, these should be averted from directly falling on the restoration until a cure is desired (less intense room lights are not a problem).

The long placement time is the biggest advantage of this type of material; there is ample opportunity to fuss with a restoration to get it exactly right before bringing in the light to cure it. At room temperature there are normally only 3 or 4 minutes to place a chemical cure restorative before it sets. However, the disadvantages of light-cured restoratives are that they must be applied in layers of 2 mm or less in order that the light can penetrate and that they need another fairly expensive piece of equipment, the light.

Types of Alternatives

▶ The Composites

The composites were invented for anterior restorations in people's mouths. They were a tremendous improvement cosmetically over amalgam or gold restorations. As far as durability is concerned, composites in the past were superior to glass ionomers, but because glass ionomers have improved, this is not necessarily the case today.

Generally what makes the composite restoration stronger is the filling material. The larger and harder the filling particles are, the stronger the material is. However, the larger particles do not finish as smooth as the small particles. Many hybrids of small and large particles are finding popularity because they compromise between good finish and strength. The one advantage composites have is that they actually swell slightly after curing to fit snugly into the tooth as they absorb the fluid in the mouth. However, regardless of type of restorative or cure, there is always microscopic shrinkage during the curing process.

With good cavity prep and undercut, a composite restoration will last for years. Composites should only be used to the level of the surface of the tooth; building them above the surface invites fracture, since there is no bond with dentin and the restoration has virtually no compressive or shearing strength. (Buildups can be made with composite or glass ionomer on nonstress surfaces if metal posts are first set into the teeth to stabilize them.) Composites do have a slight bonding with enamel, but this enamel bond is often microscopically broken during the shrinkage of curing. One of the simplest and fastest restorations to use is a chemically cured composite.

▶ *The Glass Ionomers*

Unlike the composites, acid etch and unfilled resin are used for the glass ionomers before the final material is placed. The glass ionomers also must be protected from drying with a type of varnish for about 24 hours if they are chemically cured.

The usual name for the acid that cleans the debris out of the dentinal tubules is *conditioner*. This is always rinsed off after a timed exposure (usually 15 to 30 seconds, depending on the product). Small brushes and usually a tiny tray with wells in it for the few drops of acid etch and resin (usually called *primer*) are provided with the product. The brushes are constructed of handles and disposable brush heads. Usually there are two colors of handles, and it is the technician's job to keep them straight so that the brush used for the conditioner does not find itself in the primer. You should hand the veterinarian the conditioner already in the well plus a clean brush and then dispose of the used brush immediately to prevent cross-contamination. The etched surface must be washed very thoroughly with the air/water syringe and then dried just until the surface water disappears.

The primer without filling is applied next. The primer is hydrophilic (meaning that it loves water and follows it), and the water left in the dentinal tubules induces the primer to enter the tubules to form a bond. It also allows closure of the tubules, which should mean decreased tooth sensitivity for the animal. The glass ionomer releases fluoride ions, which should increase the strength of the tooth and further dampen tooth sensitivity. Fluoride is also antimicrobial.

If the filled glass ionomer is to be mixed, it is the technician's job. You must be very precise with the tiny measured amounts; variations of the powder to resin ratio will weaken the substance and doom it to failure. The usual mixing surface is a paper pad, which can be discarded after using. The restoration is placed with instruments designed to handle this material; they are either nylon or gold tipped to keep from sticking to it and possibly coloring it. As soon as a mixed restoration hardens, it should be covered with a varnishlike material. If not, the surface will craze as it dries out. This is not true of the light-cured products, which makes them more convenient to use. However, all glass ionomers require more than one step after mixing and therefore are more involved to use than chemical-cure composites.

Alcohol can be used on instruments to clean off most nonmetal restoration materials if it is used before they set. There are additional supplies that can be helpful, such as clear Mylar strips to hold a restoration in place to prevent slumping before curing. These work even for light curing since they are clear.

After a glass ionomer restoration has solidified, it is usually shaped and polished. There are several ways to shape a tooth and restoration. One of the easiest is with a finishing bur, which has many very fine flutes (teeth) and a tapered shape to facilitate getting into the surface of the tooth. The eggbutt and flame shapes are the most often used. There are also abrasive discs, which are disposable rigid circles that snap onto a mandrel, or post, which fits into a slow-speed contra angle. The abrasive discs range from rather rough to very fine and can do a very nice job if an edge needs to be tapered flat. There are also stones and rubber discs that can be used to smooth the surface of a tooth. The tooth that carries a restoration needs to have a smooth transition between the tooth surface and the restoration because a rough edge will attract plaque and discoloration, which could even lead to caries. Certainly calculus will form more readily on a rough surface.

Client Education

One of the most valuable functions a technician can perform in a veterinary hospital is client dental education. Many times a veterinarian is tied up meeting appointments or doing procedures or other required tasks, yet the client needs personalized instruction. The ideal person to do this is you. You have the advantage of specialized knowledge combined with a hands-on, practical approach to animal care. Some clients may be nervous or overawed by the veterinarian and may relate better to you. In some cases you may be closer to the same age as the client. Also, instructing clients sharpens your communication skills and forces you to learn material, which enhances your value as an employee.

This chapter contains several invaluable handouts for the average client. Depending on the client, you may be required to explain the information in the handouts. There may also be the need to show the client how to care for his or her animal. If what is to be done is brushing teeth, and the dog has just undergone a prophy because of severe calculus and gingivitis, the time to begin brushing the dog's teeth is not now, while the gingiva is inflamed and sore. The animal's mouth should have a chance to heal before manipulating it. This would require a later appointment, perhaps incorporated into a "recheck" to see if the mouth is doing well and to elicit responses from the client about the pet's recovery, such as how much better the mouth smells or how much better the dog eats (see the form "Postprophy Questions for Clients").

Follow-up is almost always appreciated by the client and enhances the reputation of the hospital as a caring place. Even when a hospital urges people in writing to please call if they have any questions or problems, they are automatically excluding any positive comments they might hear! Plus, many people will not telephone if they think their questions are "stupid" (the most important questions to answer!). A follow-up call, if not a visit, will allow the hospital to get unsolicited compliments and to reinforce for the client how much better the pet is doing because of dental work. Or, if there are negative feelings on the part of the client that may lead to changing hospitals, the follow-up is an opportunity to deflect anger with information. The obvious person to make follow-up calls is the caring technician.

A few comments are in order for the follow-up calls. First, you should be aware of the pet's name and use it. You should review the chart before calling and have it in front of you so that you can refer to it if the owner has questions. (Personal information about the client should be appended to the file so you can establish a rapport; for instance, knowing that Mrs. Thomas prefers to be called Gladys, that her husband just died, and what special interests she might have can be used to connect more effectively with her.) A copy of the take-home instructions or a notation of the standard handouts supplied to the owner should be in the record, and the client should be asked if the information made sense (a repeated problem with a particular handout would indicate that it should be amended). Contacting the clients one week after prophies should allow them enough time to see improvement in their pets after dental care.

This questionnaire will permit the technician to discover any potential problems and to reassure the client that certain outcomes are to be expected after a prophy or extraction (especially helpful if the client has not read or understood the informational handouts).

POSTPROPHY QUESTIONS FOR CLIENTS

Questions related to anesthesia

1. Was _____ normal or was he/she depressed or lethargic after the dental cleaning? How long?
2. How soon did _____ eat after the procedure?
3. Was there any vomiting or aversion to food?
4. Does _____'s personality seem different since the procedure?

Questions related to the dental prophy

5. Is there an improvement in _____'s breath odor?
6. Does _____ chew bones, hard food, or rawhides more readily?
7. Is _____ more willing to let you handle his/her mouth?
8. Have you begun wiping or brushing the teeth? How often?

Questions related to extractions

9. Did or does _____ act as if his/her mouth is in pain?
10. Did or does _____ have blood in his/her saliva?
11. Was or is there swelling of the face or jaw after extraction?
12. How long did any swelling last?
13. Is there any bad odor associated with the mouth?

Handout 1

PROGRESSION OF PERIODONTAL DISEASE

Periodontal disease, as anyone who has read or heard advertisements for human dental products knows, is a serious illness. Periodontal disease is the establishment of bacterial infection in the mouth, infection that can travel via the bloodstream to other organs in the body.

Periodontal disease occurs in dogs and cats; it is by far the number one reason for loss of teeth in these species. In addition, it can result in mouth pain, general malaise, inappetence, and infection of other organs such as the kidneys or heart via the bloodstream. The progression of the disease occurs exactly as it does in humans (Fig. 12-1). The names of the bacteria are different in different species, but the results are the same.

Periodontal disease always begins with plaque. Plaque is the sticky, soft substance that clings to teeth and accumulates if they are not brushed or otherwise cleaned. Plaque is composed of saliva, dissolved food, bacteria, and bacterial by-products. The normal oral bacteria must have moisture and food to live in balance with the animal's immune system and to compete successfully with other microorganisms, like yeasts and fungi (yeast infections, like those caused by *Candida albicans*, typically result from antibiotic therapy that kills off normal bacteria).

Plaque is supposed to be periodically cleaned off of teeth by foodstuffs so that the bacterial numbers do not get too high. Once plaque has stayed on the teeth for a couple of days, there are millions of bacteria rapidly reproducing themselves. If there is a lot of sugar in the diet (which there often is for children but not for pets), the bacteria make excessive acid, which can eat through the enamel it contacts, resulting in caries ("cavities"). Very few pets suffer from caries. What typically happens to dogs and cats is that high numbers of bacteria and their by-products irritate the gingiva (gums) at the margin meeting the tooth, causing gingivitis. This inflammation is indicated by a red margin next to the tooth. The gingiva is the firm mound of pink tissue next to teeth. It is attached to the bone and is the first defense of the tooth root from infection. At the border of the gingiva is the oral mucosa, which lines the inside of the mouth and lips.

Plaque can and does harden to calculus ("tartar") if it is left in place on the teeth. This is because saliva contains calcium and other minerals that attach to the soft matrix. Simple chewing of food will usually not remove calculus, and brushing can seldom budge any but the softest calculus. Some chew aids for dogs and cats can be useful to remove calculus, but because calculus contains

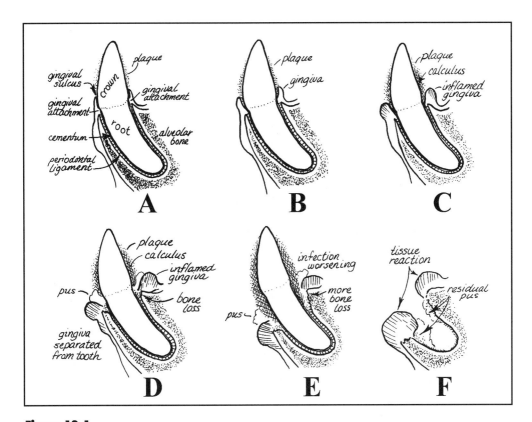

Figure 12-1

Progression of periodontal disease.

(A and B) Plaque is the inciting entity in periodontal disease. If plaque is not regularly cleaned off teeth, the bacteria it contains multiply.

(C) In addition, after about two days plaque begins to mineralize into calculus (tartar). Dental calculus is porous and contains a thriving population of bacteria; it is also mechanically irritating to soft tissues. Inflammation of the gingiva (gingivitis) with reddening and swelling is the first sign of periodontitis.

(D and E) Colonization of the gingival sulcus next to the tooth by bacteria starts the process of attachment loss because the bacteria and their by-products cause the deterioration of soft tissues and then bone.

(F) When attachment loss of the periodontal ligament reaches a certain stage, the tooth becomes loose and eventually falls out.

bacteria and protects plaque bacteria from removal, calculus tends to worsen gingivitis. It may even mechanically irritate gingiva. The result is that many animals chew less if they have gingivitis, causing the problem to get worse. Plus, because their gingivae hurt, they will refuse to allow their teeth to be brushed. If a dog or cat shows blood in saliva while chewing on a chew aid such as rawhide, it is probably from the fragile capillaries of inflamed gingiva.

Continuing to chew over a matter of days should clean the teeth and allow the gingiva to heal so that bleeding stops. However, any time bleeding is profuse or does not go away after a few days, it may be from a deep infection or a tumor, and a veterinarian should see the pet.

Gingivitis leads to more serious periodontal disease. *Periodontal* refers to structures around the teeth: the gingiva, the periodontal ligament that attaches the root of the tooth to the bone of the jaw, and the bone itself. Inflammation causes the leading edge of the gingiva to thicken and round itself, allowing plaque to be established under the gum line. Once this happens, the type of bacteria changes. The normal oral flora is aerobic, which means it thrives in the presence of air (or more specifically, oxygen). The new bacteria are anaerobic, meaning they are either killed or retarded in their growth by oxygen. The area under the gingiva is a perfect anaerobic environment.

Excessive numbers of bacteria cause oral malodor, or halitosis. The smell comes from tissues that are rotting, like spoiled meat. The odor of death and rotting is a hallmark of periodontitis.

Anaerobic bacteria are generally considered pathogenic, meaning they can cause disease. They are introduced to the mouth in small numbers on food but cause no problem unless they can find a conducive environment and reproduce in quantity. Once they are established under the gum line, they start to destroy soft tissue, like the attachment of the gingiva to the tooth and the bone and then the periodontal ligament. Finally, they even destroy bone. Often, especially in dogs, the gingiva is eaten away until there is nothing left but the mucosa that covers the bone. The mucosa, which attaches loosely rather than tightly, can not prevent bacterial invasion like healthy gingiva can. So once gingiva is lost, the tooth that it surrounds is generally doomed.

As periodontal disease worsens, pockets of infection are formed under the gingiva, which deepen as time goes on unless they are cleaned and kept clean. When they are thoroughly cleaned, the gingiva can attach back down to bone or to the tooth if the bone is gone, but this attachment is not as strong as the original. Periodontal disease can be managed but usually requires frequent cleanings, use of special treatments, and home care just to keep from worsening. Surgery on the gingiva can sometimes save teeth but tends to require heroic home care.

Unfortunately, one of the results of periodontal disease is the loss of teeth. Infection progresses along the root until either the attached gingiva is gone in one or more places around the tooth or enough bone and periodontal ligament are destroyed that the tooth is loose and acting as a painful foreign body in the mouth. Teeth affected in this way are sources of infection and distress for the animal, and it is cruel to insist on saving them until they fall out.

Dogs and cats can and do thrive without teeth, even if they are eating only dry food. Commercial animal diets have been processed into bite-sized pieces that merely require swallowing. Most dogs and cats with severe periodontal disease have not been chewing on the affected teeth because it is so painful, but once gingivae have healed after extractions, they will often chew vigorously, even with toothless jaws. After thorough cleaning and extractions cats and dogs tend to feel so much better that many owners say their pets have a new lease on life. The lack of offensive mouth odor also makes them much more enjoyable company.

Handout 2

CLEANING YOUR PET'S TEETH

To prevent the progression of periodontal disease, it is important to keep plaque off the teeth on a regular basis. Studies have shown that without dental care most dogs and cats show at least the beginnings of periodontal disease by age 3. Since periodontal disease is so much easier to prevent than to manage, it is important that pets be started as early as possible with home dental care.

For many pets, home dental care relies mostly on brushing. Although there are diets that can reduce plaque and calculus (such as Hill's Science Diet [Canine and Feline t/d] and Friskies Dental Diet), some pets may not find them palatable, and the teeth they clean off are usually the rear cutting and grinding teeth only. Chew aids, like rawhide, ropes, artificial bones, and toys, tend to only work on dogs' rear teeth, cannot do any good if the animals refuse to use them, and may even be dangerous to their teeth. For dogs, fractures of teeth not related to traumatic accidents are most frequently caused by chewing narrow, hard artificial bones, narrow pieces of real bone, and "chew hooves." The dangerous width seems to be between ¼ and ½ in.; when dogs get these hard substances between the two large carnassial teeth in the back of their mouths, they fracture off a slab of one of the teeth. The best of the chew aids is rawhide in a simple chip form. It is most like what an animal would consume in the wild, where the elastic fibers of tendons, ligaments, fibrous tissue in the muscle, or skin stretch over teeth to wipe off the plaque as teeth perforate them. However, some dogs rapidly chew off big chunks of the rawhide, or swallow them whole, which can lead to intestinal obstruction or simply vomiting them in the house. So in the final analysis, brushing is the only sure protection for pet teeth.

It is easier to train a dog or cat from puppy- or kittenhood than to begin with an older animal, but either can be accomplished. One thing that is important for an adult animal is not to begin trying to brush if the animal already has signs of gingivitis. If the gums are reddened, or if there is already calculus (tartar) present, there will be discomfort when the brush goes over the soft tissue. This animal's teeth should be professionally cleaned before brushing is begun because brushing will not remove calculus and will only teach the animal to fight the procedure because it hurts.

Training follows a simple, stepwise plan. First, the animal is accustomed to having fingers rubbed under lips and in cheeks against the teeth. As soon as the animal holds still (even a little bit) for this manipulation, he or she is rewarded, even if the reward is only praise or petting. Small food treats work

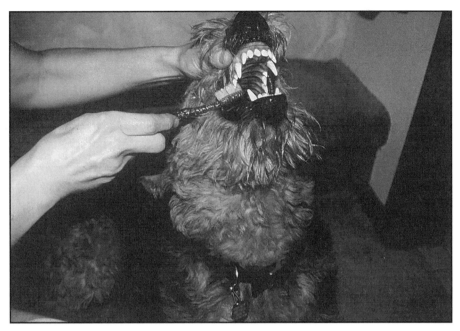

Figure 12-2
Brushing teeth can be a fun experience for both owner and dog.

well with dogs, but the food needs to be given immediately after the correct behavior to be effective and should never be given within 10 minutes if he or she was naughty and did not do what you wanted. The goal is to get the animal to hold still while you handle his or her mouth as long and extensively as you want. How the mouth is opened is also important for dogs. To do this, you press your thumb against the lip over the upper teeth midway from eye to nose as you hold your fingers over the muzzle. When the dog opens his or her mouth, you hold your thumb on the roof of the mouth; the dog will keep his or her mouth open and will not bite down but will probably pull away. You get the dog to increase the time of leaving his or her mouth open by praise and reward (Fig. 12-2).

If the pet readily accepts your fingers in his or her mouth, the next stage is to wipe something over the teeth. It can be a washcloth, gauze, or even a finger cot brush. There are some animals that never progress beyond the wiping stage, but ideally you want to introduce the brush and do a more thorough job of removing plaque. The brush should be as soft as possible; smaller children's toothbrushes or special brushes for dogs and cats can be used. The act of brushing is more important than the dentifrice (toothpaste) because the mechanical movement, not the toothpaste, removes the plaque. Human

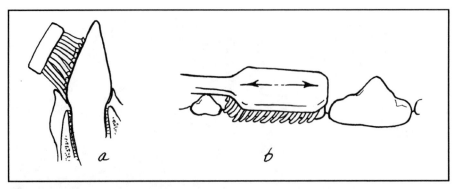

Figure 12-3
Since dog teeth in general are not close together like those of people, the most important area to clean is the crown of the tooth next to the gingiva on the outside of the teeth (a). (The tongue tends to keep the insides of the teeth clean.) This can be accomplished by a simple back-and-forth brushing (b) with the brush angled into the gingival sulcus.

toothpaste should not be used on pets because it is designed to be spat out, and swallowing it can cause stomach upset. Animal toothpastes are designed to be very palatable to pets, and toothpaste can be a reward to pets for allowing brushing. However, toothpaste is not necessary for clean teeth. The brush may be used alone or with salt, garlic salt (which dogs like), or baking soda (unless the animal is on a salt-restricted diet).

The areas that are most subject to plaque are the outsides of the teeth because the tongue tends to keep plaque cleaned off of the insides. However, some small dogs are prone to periodontitis on the insides of the upper canines, so these areas should be brushed by holding the mouth open. Remember to brush around the corner in the upper back of the mouth where periodontitis often begins. It is generally not necessary to use an up-and-down motion since most pet teeth are not close together like human teeth. The brush should be held against the teeth at about a 45-degree angle toward the gums, and the brush moved back and forth across the teeth (Fig. 12-3). The major area where plaque accumulates is near the gum line, and pressing the toothbrush against the teeth will even allow the bristles to go somewhat between the teeth at this level.

Daily toothbrushing of pets is ideal, but brushing will usually be effective if done at least twice a week. The reason for this is that it normally takes two to three days for bacterial numbers in plaque to increase enough to cause gingivitis. Brushing a pet's teeth infrequently is often not only ineffective but it will cause aversion to brushing because the pet has gingivitis.

Cats can be very uncooperative about brushing, and you may be forced to take them more often to the veterinary hospital to get their teeth cleaned. A couple of hints for training cats: There are very few food treats that cats will work for, although there are some that are attractive to most cats and some individual special treats that most cats crave, such as Pounce and Purina Whisker Lickins. It is always an excellent idea to trim the toenails of all four feet before embarking on something a cat may not like, like toothbrushing. Also, the small size of the cat's mouth makes brushing difficult from a mechanical point of view, so it may pay to get a brush specially made for cats.

Handout 3

DENTAL CARE RECOMMENDATIONS FOR PETS

The average dog or cat will already show signs of periodontal disease by the age of 3; some unfortunate individuals will have problems even earlier. Pure-bred cats and small-breed dogs seem to be the most susceptible, which indicates there is a breed and a size component. Regular visits with the veterinarian will help you to know if your animal needs professional attention, but you can judge yourself if the animal may need teeth-cleaning maintenance. It is time to have the teeth cleaned if the gingival (gum) margins next to the teeth are reddened, if the teeth are obviously discolored by calculus (tartar), or if the animal's breath smells of decay or rotting.

Manipulating the pet's mouth from early on should be a goal of every pet owner. Early handling will help in training for brushing (see the handout "Cleaning Your Pet's Teeth"). If you are not willing to spend regular time brushing teeth, you should be prepared to schedule frequent teeth cleanings at the veterinary hospital. The alternative may be pain, loss of teeth, and long-standing infection.

Chew aids may help keep an animal's teeth clean. "Oral" breeds of dog, such as retrievers, often keep their teeth clean just because they are constantly chewing on things. Many never need to have their teeth cleaned, and although their teeth may be worn down, they tend to keep all their teeth throughout their lifetime. Good chew aids for dogs include rawhide, some rope toys, and large, fresh bones. Chew toys that probably don't affect dental health include rubber figures, balls, and most biscuits. Items that can be very bad for dogs, because they break teeth, are cows' hooves, narrow natural bones, and narrow, hard plastic bones—in fact, any hard substance between ¼ and ½ in. wide that a dog will chew.

Dry food is generally better than canned food, not because it cleans teeth (there are only a small number of special diets designed to actually clean teeth as the animal chews) but because the food does not get as readily dissolved in the saliva to provide food for bacteria in the plaque. Similarly, hard biscuits usually just crack apart when chewed and do not scrape the sides of the teeth to clean them. Recently, appetizing and nutritious dog and cat food and treats designed to clean teeth have been introduced. If effective, these may prove useful for self-dental cleaning in cats, who are notorious for not cooperating with brushing.

Handout 4

FELINE STOMATITIS

Cats are subject to an often exquisitely painful condition called stomatitis, which means inflammation of the mouth. This syndrome is actually an extensive type of periodontitis, where not only the gingival (gum) and other periodontal tissues are involved but also the lining of the throat, cheeks, lips, and sometimes tongue. No one knows what exactly causes feline stomatitis, but it apparently has a bacterial and an allergic component to it. Some cats are susceptible to it while others are not.

The bacteria that initiate stomatitis are those that cause periodontitis. When the cat has a clean, healthy mouth, stomatitis is held at bay. As soon as bacteria start increasing, however, the animal mounts an allergic reaction to the bacteria and/or their metabolites (those substances the bacteria make and release into the environment), which spreads to nearby structures. The bacteria have only one spot that is protected enough to proliferate in the mouth: the dental sulcus. The sulcus is the area between the flap of gingiva over the tooth and the tooth itself. The sulcus is deepened into a periodontal pocket as bacteria increase, but sometimes periodontitis is not very advanced when the cat's body becomes sensitive to the bacteria.

Stomatitis often occurs only in the rear of the mouth, leaving the front teeth, the canines (or fangs), and the incisors (the small teeth between the canines) relatively unaffected. Characteristic of stomatitis is bright red gingiva and mucosa (the lining of the cheek and the back of the mouth). Typically, the mucosa is very fragile and is covered by a slimy layer of saliva and reactive white blood cells. When sections of this tissue are submitted for microscopic analysis and are found to be full of lymphocytes and plasma cells (white blood cells involved in producing antibodies against foreign substances), the cat has what pathologists call lymphocytic/plasmacytic stomatitis.

Treatment of stomatitis first involves cleaning the teeth and keeping them clean. Then antibiotics or oral disinfectants may be used to keep down the numbers of bacteria. Finally antiinflammatory agents (usually corticosteroids) may be given as a last attempt at medical treatment. Sometimes the condition will respond to cleaning alone, or cleaning with oral disinfectants, and so on. Often the veterinarian goes through the entire list of treatments unsuccessfully, or what once worked becomes ineffective. Treatment with drugs (steroids particularly) can damage the liver if given for long periods. Unfortunately, the condition often resists treatment, or it resurfaces, and the cat is in so much pain that he or she cannot eat, with oral pain resulting in constant salivation. When the condition has proved intractable, the veterinarian is forced to use the final solution: extracting the teeth that are allowing the bacteria to proliferate.

If the condition is confined to the rear of the mouth, extracting only the caudal teeth may allow the cat to return to oral health. At any rate, extraction of the front teeth can be done at a later date if the first procedure is not curative. For the worst case a whole-mouth extraction must be performed. This must be done carefully so that no root fragments are left behind to cause sore areas. The result will be a toothless but comfortable cat.

Handout 5

RESORPTIVE LESIONS OF FELINE TEETH

There is a unique syndrome in cats in which cells from the bone eat away teeth. Certain bone cells called osteoclasts are constantly eating tunnels through the bone. Following them closely are other cells called osteoblasts that fill in the tunnel with new bone, and the new bone is called an osteoid seam. The constant renewal of bone keeps it strong and responsive to stresses put on it. Osteoclasts occur throughout the bone, so they also are in the bone of the tooth socket next to the gingiva. For some reason, when inflammation occurs where the gingiva (gums) meets the tooth and the bony socket in cats, there is sometimes a mobilization of the osteoclasts from the bone to attack the tooth where the enamel covering the dentin of the crown meets the dentin of the root.

Osteoclasts have no trouble eating away dentin; the dentin of the tooth is a dense modified bone. Amazingly, this process can proceed so rapidly that a tooth can be lost in a few weeks or months. As the osteoclasts eat away the dentin, the osteoblasts do not follow them, and a concavity is produced. Resorptive lesions are classed 1, 2, or 3, according to how much of the tooth is destroyed.

Class 1 resorptive lesions just barely invade the surface of the tooth. They usually cannot be seen, but their edges can be felt with a metal dental explorer. Class 2 lesions are obvious defects that can be both seen and felt. However, they have not perforated the pulp. Class 3 lesions have invaded the pulp. Deep lesions often proceed until a large portion of the tooth crowns and roots is eaten away. Radiographs (X rays) of these teeth often show them as hollow shells. As the strength of the tooth crowns is diminished, these teeth tend to snap off at the gum line, often leaving sharp shards of the roots underneath the gingiva. These sharp ends can cause sores in the mouth and are usually painful to chew on.

A hallmark of resorptive lesions, especially classes 2 and 3, is their painfulness. Cats may paw at their mouths, avoid their faces being touched, refuse food, or salivate profusely in response to resorptive lesions. Even when cats are anesthetized, their jaws will "chatter" when the lesions are touched. The reason they are so painful is that first the dentinal insulation for the nerves of the pulp is reduced, and then it is absent altogether. Resorptive lesions most often occur between the roots of the more forward cheek teeth, but they can occur anywhere in the mouth, wherever periodontal inflammation happens. Since periodontitis usually starts on the "outside" of the mouth (because the tongue tends to keep the inside of the teeth cleaner than the outside), most resorptive lesions are along the gum line on the sides of the mouth. Often, the gingiva responds to class 2 and class 3 resorptive lesions by filling in the hole with a bright red bleb of soft tissue. This tissue probably acts like a Band-Aid over the raw nerves.

Feline resorptive lesions were originally called cat cavities, which is a very catchy but incorrect name. *Cavity* is a common term for caries in people. Caries is bacterial destruction of enamel and dentin. It is characterized by dark, soft-walled, rotten dentin. Feline resorptive lesions are clean and hard edged. Because *dentin* is devoured, another name for these is feline *odonto-clastic* resorptive lesions. They have also been known as cervical line lesions because they begin at the junction of the root and crown, which is known as the neck (or cervix) of the tooth. By any name they are bad news for the cat.

Treatment for these lesions, if they are painful, is usually extraction. If the lesion extends into the pulp, there is no saving the tooth because it is significantly weakened and the endodontal system of cats is too small to do root canals except in the canine teeth. Class 1 and class 2 lesions may be filled with dental restoratives. Unfortunately, many of these fail because of osteoclasts renewing their attack in the same area. One study found only 20 percent of restorations were in place after 18 months.

If retained roots have healthy pink gingiva over them and are not found to be painful when probed while the cat is lightly anesthetized, they may be left in place. If there are sores over the roots, or if pressing them causes a response, they should be removed.

Fortunately, only a portion of the cat population is susceptible to resorptive lesions and usually only a few teeth are affected.

Handout 6

POSTANESTHESIA CARE FOR PETS

Special home care is needed by animals that have been released on the same day they have been under general anesthesia for dental procedures or surgery. Many pets are more sedate for several hours after anesthesia due to lingering effects of the drugs. Some may even appear slightly "drunk," especially when they first arise after resting. You should be ready for this loss of balance and assist your pet into and out of your vehicle, up or down stairs, and onto and off of furniture to prevent an accidental fall. It is not unusual for grogginess to persist for 24 hours or more after anesthesia, but the animal should become progressively more alert rather than more depressed during the recovery period.

Because a pet may be disoriented during the postanesthesia period, we recommend that you provide a confined and quiet area for him or her to sleep it off. Other pets should not be allowed to pester or harm the recovering animal, and small children should be prevented from startling or bothering the recovering pet and possibly getting bitten or scratched.

Since animals recovering from anesthesia may not adequately control their body temperature, they should not be expected to tolerate extremes of environmental temperature, especially cold, for 24 hours after anesthesia. Even animals accustomed to living outside should not be left in an unheated environment on a cold night after anesthesia.

Older animals, who often have compromised kidney function, are given intravenous (IV) fluids during the anesthesia period. This generally provides enough fluid for kidney function for several hours after anesthesia. However, if the animal is denied water, the kidneys can be damaged, so it is important that normal water consumption be resumed as soon as possible after anesthesia. After 10 or 12 hours postanesthesia, refusal to drink water or inability to tolerate water in the stomach (vomiting) can be a sign of serious anesthesia side effects of which we should be made aware. Because anesthesia causes nausea and vomiting in some animals, food should first be offered in small quantities only after an animal has completely recovered equilibrium. If the animal has not vomited by one hour after feeding, a full meal may be provided. Please call if you have any questions about water or food consumption after anesthesia.

Some animals may have tracheal (windpipe) irritation from the tube used to deliver the gas anesthetic, resulting in a soft cough. This will usually resolve in a few days without treatment. If a cough persists, if an animal does not seem normal within a day of returning home, if he or she should seem to get more quiet or depressed over time rather than more awake, or if you should have any other concerns, please call the hospital. Even at night, personnel are available to help your pet.

Handout 7

DENTAL EXTRACTIONS

Extractions of teeth in pets may be required for several reasons, including deep-seated infection due to periodontal disease, resorptive lesions in cats, and fractures with infections of the endodontal system (the pulp of the tooth) in which root canal therapy is not desired or not possible. Periodontal disease is by far the main reason for loss of teeth in pets. Extraction will provide relief from pain and infection for teeth that cannot be saved.

Extracting teeth that are irretrievably affected involves some postextraction pain, but much of this can be controlled by drugs. Even before pain medications were widespread, some animals would be in less pain immediately after extractions than before because loose teeth in infected gingiva and bone would cause pain every time the mouth was closed. In general, because the mouth has such a good blood supply, healing after extractions is very rapid. Many times extraction sites can be sutured, which speeds healing and is usually less painful for the animal, but it is not appropriate to suture all extraction sites. Often the gingiva is so fragile due to infection that it will not hold a suture, or infection is so deep and widespread that the site is left open to drain. Some extraction sites are so tiny that the clot that forms in the socket is adequate to allow healing. Sutures used in the mouth are absorbable so that they do not have to be removed. They may be present many weeks past the time when the gingiva is completely healed, but they do not cause any problems by being there.

Many animals have blood in their saliva for two to three days after extractions. This is totally normal during the healing process as the pet eats, chews a toy, or otherwise bumps the extraction site. If bleeding should continue more than this period, or if bleeding is profuse, the pet should be seen by a veterinarian. You should be prepared for possible light bleeding from the mouth by keeping the pet away from anything you don't want permanently stained.

Depending on the extent of infection and inflammation, antibiotics and perhaps antiinflammatories may be dispensed for your pet after extractions. These will speed healing and reduce discomfort in cases for which they are appropriate, and they should be given as directed.

Worries that a dog or cat won't be able to eat after extractions are unfounded. Pet foods are processed so that a pet doesn't need teeth at all, even for dry diets. The small kibbles can be swallowed whole without any digestive problems in most pets, and even without teeth many animals will chew dry food once the gums heal. In general we do not recommend that the diet be changed to canned food after extractions, unless the pet refuses regular dry food. This is because there sometimes are digestive upsets (such as gas or diarrhea) with diet change and because the pet may resist changing back to the normal diet. After all, if there were only a few extractions, the pet did not chew on those painful teeth before they were extracted nor will he or she chew on tender extraction sites. If, however, the pet refuses to eat a regular dry diet, the kibbles can be made soft by adding an approximately equal amount of water about 30 minutes before feeding.

During your pet's dental extractions he or she was under general anesthesia. We may have also used a local anesthetic, but it would have been limited by where the tooth is located. We try to avoid local anesthesia that will deaden the tongue or lips because the pet can gnaw on these without realizing it. To prevent serious trauma, we would like to know immediately if your pet appears to be chewing on tongue or lips.

Local anesthesia is intended to reduce postextraction pain. We also administer analgesics (pain killers) at the hospital, which may cause drowsiness when the animal goes home, and either dispense pain medication or recommend over-the-counter painkillers. In general, 12 to 24 hours after extraction is the most painful period, and pain medications should be continued for that period at least. Specific instructions about drugs to be given to your pet for pain or infection will be on your dismissal form.

Handout 8

FRACTURED AND TRAUMATIZED TEETH

Dogs and cats frequently break teeth. In cats the occasion for tooth fracture is usually falling or being hit by a car. Dogs tend to have more of a variety of accidents, including being hit by a car, being kicked by a horse or cow, catching a rock instead of ball, and so on. Dogs also are prone to breaking teeth by chewing the wrong thing. Many dogs that are kept in wire kennels or restrained by wire fences will often pull at the wire with their canine teeth. This wears a groove in the back of the teeth over time, weakening them. Then one time when they grab the wire, a tooth snaps off. Teeth of these "fence biters" will fracture more readily than those of other dogs in other situations when teeth are stressed. A dog that is not accustomed to being kenneled may get normal teeth caught in wire as he or she jumps up to escape and will snap off canines, incisors, or even premolars.

Other dogs fracture rear teeth chewing on inappropriate substances, some of which are offered to them by their owners. The usual victims are the upper carnassial teeth. The carnassial teeth are the large teeth in the back of the upper and lower jaws that are used in a scissors action to cut through meat. You will notice that a dog will chew with these teeth when he or she has something tough to reduce to bite-sized pieces. The problem is that narrow, hard substances, when chewed between these teeth, tend to snap off a slab of the upper carnassial tooth. A large dog can exert a thousand pounds per square inch of pressure with his or her jaws, and the pressure is greatest when the jaws are nearly closed. The most dangerous thickness seems to be between ¼ to ½ in. (6–11 mm). The most common items to cause these fractures are dried cow hooves, hard plastic artificial bones (both of which are commonly sold as chewing toys by pet stores), and narrow bones, such as from steaks. Obviously, the fracture of the carnassial is due to a mechanical wedge effect, and the wedge does not have to be as strong as a tooth, just fairly firm and resistant to compression. Occasionally dogs neurotically chew on rocks or metal and fracture teeth.

Dogs, particularly puppies that are "teething," often enjoy gnawing on bones or other substances. Bones, when provided to dogs, should be of a large diameter and dense, such as the joint and leg bones of cattle. Dogs should be started as puppies with bones so that they learn how hard to chew on dense substances. Bones should be removed as soon as they become shards or splinters. Not only can the small pieces break teeth, but they can lodge in any area of the digestive tract, necessitating surgery (the reason chicken bones should never be fed to dogs). Or the dog can simply vomit them up on your carpet.

Rawhide is a better chew aid for most dogs; it is never hard enough to break teeth. Still, a dog that swallows it whole is not getting the value for his or her teeth, and it is likely to make the dog vomit or to cause obstruction in the digestive tract.

A fracture of the tooth can be either open or closed. These terms refer to the pulp of the tooth. The pulp, or endodontal system, contains blood and lymph vessels, nerves, cells that produce dentin, and cells that provide the support tissue for the other structures. Because the nerves are exposed in an open fracture, the first response is pain, especially when air contacts it. Any person who has had an open tooth fracture can attest to this.

A fresh open fracture is an emergency. The life of the tooth can be saved, and pain instantly relieved, if a procedure called a pulp cap or vital pulpotomy is performed. In this procedure, a small amount of contaminated pulp is removed, a dressing of calcium hydroxide is placed over the pulp, and the pulp chamber is sealed with a restoration (filling). The pet is usually sent home with antibiotics, which will take care of any bacteria that may still be in the tooth. A pulp cap must be performed immediately, generally within 24 hours of the fracture. You can tell if a fracture is fresh because the pulp will be actively bleeding or there will be a red dot of pulp on the tooth. Signs of pain are salivation, pawing at the mouth, reluctance or refusing to eat or drink cold water, or crying out when chewing. Some dogs are very stoic and do not demonstrate any signs of there being something wrong; these should be very carefully examined if oral trauma is suspected.

What happens if you do not notice when the animal broke the tooth and weeks or months elapse? The bacteria that merely contaminated the tip of the pulp begin to infect it. Bacterial invasion induces the body to send white blood cells to fight the infection, and small blood vessels dilate and become leaky to fluid. The result is the swelling of inflammation. Since the swelling is within an unyielding structure (the tooth dentin), it presses on the nerves, causing pain. This condition is called pulpitis.

Infection in the pulp will eventually reach the apex of the root. Multirooted teeth have communication between the pulp chambers of each root at the level of the crown. When the infection leaves the root, it first destroys the periodontal ligament and then attacks the bone of the socket. This early bone infection is exceedingly painful; this is a tooth root abscess. The bone tries to seal off the infection with new bone, but if the infection is overwhelming, it simply continues to eat bone until it can find a way out, forming an abscess tract into the mouth, out the side of the face, or into nose or sinus. The swollen face or draining tract usually becomes evident about six to eight weeks after the fracture, but it can potentially occur as long as the tooth is left untreated, even if the bone has initially sealed it. Usually by the time a draining tract is formed, the majority of the pain is over. Occasionally the infection can be cleared by antibiotics, but it almost always comes back because there is a reservoir of bacteria in the tooth that will reactivate once the antibiotics are gone.

Judging by the large numbers of old fractures seen without clinical signs in dogs, the majority of open fractures are sealed off by bone. Unfortunately, before that happened, the animal suffered in silence.

The only way to effect a permanent cure is with endodontal therapy, specifically a root canal. A root canal consists of cleaning the pulp chamber thoroughly with tiny round files, disinfecting it, and then filling it with a combination of inert filler and a cement that will kill any remaining bacteria. The fracture hole and any other access holes for the root canal are filled with a restoration to complete the process. Immature teeth, in which the root tip has not closed off, require a procedure called apexification before a root canal can be performed because the cement used in the root canal can cause irritation to the bone if the root apex is still open.

Any tooth that has died due to infection, or has undergone a root canal, is more brittle than it was when it was alive. Owners need to protect their investment in root canal therapy by keeping dogs from chewing or biting hard substances. Dogs that chew rocks are poor candidates for root canal therapy because they will probably break the tooth that has had a root canal. The tooth should probably be extracted instead.

Some fractured teeth cannot be saved by pulp cap or root canal procedures. A fracture that extends from the crown into the root will not allow a seal between pulp and mouth, and a fractured or resorbed (eaten away) root will not provide a seal between pulp and bone. These teeth should be extracted.

Some fractures do not require any therapy at all. A closed fracture, in which enamel or enamel and dentin are chipped but the pulp is not exposed, does not need to be treated. The tooth will be more sensitive to cold than normal because the enamel and dentin act as insulation. However, if the tooth is alive, it will manufacture more dentin to protect the pulp. Closed fractures may benefit from fluoride treatment because fluoride reduces sensitivity and strengthens tooth structure.

Teeth that have suffered trauma but that do not have broken crowns may become discolored. This is because blood has been released from the small blood vessels in the tooth pulp just as it is in a bruise on your body. The red blood cells disintegrate outside of the blood vessels, and the hemoglobin passes into the dentin, coloring it pinkish or purple. If the teeth are alive, the color will often gradually fade. If the teeth are dead, the color will not only not fade but it may also turn grayish. A gray/black tooth is almost certainly dead.

The ideal treatment for a dead tooth, whether it is a bruised tooth or a sound one with an old open fracture, is a root canal. If there are no clinical signs of abscessation, pain, or swelling, the owners may prefer to "wait and see," realizing, of course, that there is always the potential for a dead tooth to abscess. If an abscess is present, the tooth should have a root canal or be extracted immediately.

Handout 9

THE ROOT CANAL

Root canals are most often used for fractured teeth that are devitalized, infected, or dead. Sometimes a tooth has abscessed, meaning infection from the tooth has exited the tooth at the root apex and infected the bone. This abscess is repaired by a root canal.

The procedure for a root canal is to create access to the pulp, sometimes through a fracture and sometimes through another access site that allows better exposure to the root pulp. The pulp canal is then cleaned of any soft pulp or necrotic debris remaining in it by use of tiny round files. After disinfection, the pulp is then packed tightly with a combination of a cement with a latex-like substance called gutta percha. Finally, the tooth pulp is sealed off with a restoration (filling). The root canal prevents infection in the bone because the filling of gutta percha and cement will not support the growth of bacteria. During the root canal, X rays are taken to ensure that the pulp chamber has been filled.

Most root canals in dogs and cats are a complete success, but problems are not unknown. A dead tooth (one without a living, functioning pulp) is more brittle than a live tooth and is more subject to fracture. If a tooth is rebroken, bacteria may enter from the mouth and result in an apical abscess. If bacteria are still present in the apex of the root, they can result in an abscess. Abscesses may show as pain or reluctance to bite down on the affected tooth or as swellings or draining tracts on the face or chin above or under the root tip.

Owners need to monitor the restoration in the tooth and make sure it is intact at the surface of the tooth and not depressed or showing signs of leakage (a dark line or crevice around the restoration). Also, X rays of the tooth should be taken when the animal has the regular teeth cleaning to ensure that the root canal is still functioning to seal the pulp chamber.

Handout 10

AFTERCARE FOR PULP CAPS
(VITAL PULPOTOMIES)

If your pet has suffered a fresh fracture of a tooth, the treatment of choice is often the pulp cap. The pulp cap (a.k.a. vital pulpotomy) can save the life and strength of the tooth. The live part of the tooth is the vital pulp in the center of the tooth. This tissue consists of cells that make dentin, the hard substance of the tooth under the thin layer of enamel; blood and lymph vessels; nerves; and cells and fibers that support the rest of the structures. The pulp has no capacity to heal itself, like skin does, so if it is exposed to the bacteria in the mouth, it will become infected and eventually die.

An infected tooth can result in infection in the bone (an apical abscess). When the pulp is alive, exposure of the tooth's nerve causes pain. When the pulp dies, the tooth becomes brittle and therefore not as strong. Because of short- and long-term problems, it is best to treat fractures of teeth immediately with pulp caps.

The pulp cap consists of taking out a few millimeters of contaminated pulp, placing a dressing into the pulp chamber on the remaining pulp, and then packing a restoration, or filling, to the outside surface of the tooth. The dressing is calcium hydroxide, which stimulates the pulp to make more dentin under the restoration and which also is a potent antibacterial substance. The result for the animal is immediate cessation of pain because there is no longer exposure of the pulp to the air.

Because of the exposure of the pulp to bacteria, we send animals home with antibiotics to help the body destroy any remaining bacteria the pulp may contain. Because bacteria have access to the pulp, and because the blood supply to the pulp may have been damaged in a traumatic accident leading to the death of the tooth, we like to see the dog or cat back for X rays after four months. This will allow us to see if new dentin is being laid down under the restoration or if there is an abscess at the root tip because the tooth died and became infected. (Death and infection of the tooth may result in the tooth requiring a root canal or extraction.)

The outlook for the tooth after a pulp cap depends on several things. One is the amount of bacterial contamination. A dog with a very dirty mouth that has periodontitis present will have a poorer prognosis than a dog with a clean mouth. The length of time since the tooth was broken will determine how long the pulp was exposed to bacteria and how much of a foothold they could get. A young dog has much more blood circulation than an older dog; the increased circulation is useful for fighting infection. As mentioned above, trauma to the tooth can impair the circulation; this impairment may not be evident at the time of performing the pulp cap.

Pulp caps are used when crowns are amputated into the pulp, as they are when teeth are damaging tissues, are interfering with other teeth, or need to be taken off in order to prevent aggressive dogs from leaving deep bite wounds. Because of the ability to control cleanliness, a crown amputation with a pulp cap generally has a better prognosis than a pulp cap on a tooth that has been traumatically fractured.

It is very important to check the restoration regularly. If the restoration should come out or leak around the edges, bacteria may infect the pulp. Marginal leakage will show as a dark line on the edges of the restoration. Dogs that are vigorous chewers may implode the restoration into the tooth, creating leakage around it; this may show only as the restoration being slightly below the tooth surface where it began. If the pulp infection should turn into an abscess, the animal may show signs of mouth pain, such as reluctance to bite down with that tooth.

Abscesses occasionally present as soft tissue swellings on the face or jaw, which may turn into draining tracts. They originate at the root tips, so swellings for the upper fourth premolar (carnassial tooth) would appear under the eye, for the upper canine midway between eye and nose just below the bridge of the nose, and for the lower canine about the same area from front to back except under the affected side of the jaw.

Related Books

Some general small animal dentistry texts published after 1990:

2000   D.H. DeForge and B.H. Colmery III, eds. *An Atlas of Veterinary Dental Radiology*. Ames: Iowa State University Press.

1999   J. Bellows. *The Practice of Veterinary Dentistry: A Team Effort*. Ames: Iowa State University Press.

1999   F.J.M. Verstraete, ed. *Self-Assessment Color Review of Veterinary Dentistry*. Ames: Iowa State University Press.

1998   S.E. Holmstrom, ed. *Canine Dentistry*, Veterinary Clinics of North America (Small Animal Practice) 28:5. Philadelphia: WB Saunders.

1998   S.E. Holmstrom, P. Frost, E.R. Eisner. *Veterinary Dental Techniques for the Small Animal Practitioner* (2nd ed.). Philadelphia: WB Saunders.

1997   R.B. Wiggs and H.B. Lobprise. *Veterinary Dentistry: Principles and Practice*. Philadelphia: Lippincott-Raven.

1995   D.A. Crossley and S. Penman, eds. 1995. *Manual of Small Animal Dentistry* (2nd ed.). Ames: Iowa State University Press.

1993   E.C. Harvey and P.P. Emily. *Small Animal Dentistry*. St. Louis: Mosby.

1993   P. Kertesz. *A Colour Atlas of Veterinary Dentistry and Oral Surgery*. London: Wolfe (Mosby—Year Book Europe, Ltd.).

1992   A.D. Shipp and P. Fahrenkrug. *Practitioners' Guide to Veterinary Dentistry*. Beverly Hills, Calif.: Dr. Shipp's Laboratories.

1990   P. Emily and E. Penman. *Handbook of Small Animal Dentistry*. Oxford: Pergamon.

Veterinary Dental Associations

Academy of Veterinary Dentistry (AVD)

The AVD is an accrediting association for veterinary dentists. Veterinarians who qualify by experience and examination become fellows of the academy.

American Society of Veterinary Dental Technicians (ASVDT)

The society provides training materials and accredits veterinary dental technicians.

P.O. Box 1636
Venice, Florida 34284-1636

American Veterinary Dental College (AVDC)

Like other specialty boards within the American Veterinary Medical Association (AVMA), the college maintains a training program and qualifying examination for membership for graduate veterinarians or dentists.

American Veterinary Dental Society (AVDS)

The AVDS publishes the *Journal of Veterinary Dentistry*. The journal subscription is included in the annual membership fee ($60). Membership is open.

Walker Management Group (WMG)

The WMG is a central information resource for the American Veterinary Dental Society, the Academy of Veterinary Dentistry, and the American Veterinary Dental College as well as the national veterinary dental meeting, Veterinary Dental Forum, sponsored by these three organizations.

Walker Management Group/Veterinary Dentistry
530 Church Street, Suite 700
Nashville, Tennessee 37219
(800) 254-3687 Information
(615) 344-7333 Fax

Dental Abbreviations of the American Veterinary Dental College

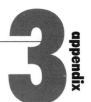

Category[a]	Abbreviation	Meaning
PA	AB	Abrasion
P	CI3	Abundance of supra- or subgingival calculus
P	P3	Abundant soft material in sulcus
S	ACY	Acrylic
PAX	OM-ADC	Adenocarcinoma
P	AP	Alveoloplasty
O	AXB	Anterior cross-bite
E	APX	Apexification
E	APG	Apexogenesis
G	A	Apical
E	AS	Apical sealer/cement
PX	AL	Attachment loss
P	PD1	0% Attachment loss (AL)—gingivitis
P	PD3	25–50% Attachment loss
PA	AT	Attrition
PAX	EP/B	Basal cell carcinoma (acanthomatous)
PA	BE	Biopsy, excisional
S	BE	Biopsy, excisional
S	BI	Biopsy, incisional
PA	BI	Biopsy, incisional
O	TRANS	Body movement or translation
P	BG	Bone graft
P	BL	Bone loss or recession
O	MAL 2	Brachygnathia
O	BKT	Bracket
O	T	Bracket marked on chart
RX	BR	Bridge
RX	BRC	Bridge, cantilever
RX	BRM	Bridge, Maryland
RX	BP	Bridge, pontic
G	B	Buccal
S	BFR	Buccal fold removal
PAX	CAL	Calculus
PX	CAL	Calculus
PAX	CI	Calculus index

Category[a]	Abbreviation	Meaning
P	CI	Calculus index (Ramfjord)
R	CA	Cavity
RX	CA	Cavity, fracture or defect (1–8)
RX	C/MOD	Cavity, mesial occlusal distal surface
PA	O	Circle around missing tooth on chart
S	CFW	Circumferential wiring
P	CT	Citric acid treatment
RX	C1N	Class I, pulp exposure, nonvital
RX	C1V	Class I, pulp exposure, vital
S	CFL	Cleft lip
S	CFP	Cleft palate
S	CFP/R	Cleft palate repair
P	RPC	Closed root planing
P	PRO	Complete prophylaxis
PX	CU	Contact ulcer (kissing ulcer)
R	CBU	Core buildup
G	C	Coronal/cuspid
PAX	CMO	Craniomandibular osteopathy
O	MAL 1	Cross-bite (jaw relation normal)
PAX	CWD	Crowding
R	CR	Crown
E	CAM	Crown, amputation, reduction
R	CMB	Crown, base metal
R	CMG	Crown, gold metal
R	RS	Crown lost, root tips remain
R	CM	Crown, metal
R	PFM	Crown, porcelain fused to metal
M	CUL	Culture
M	CS	Culture/sensitivity
RX	C6	Cusp
PAX	DC	Cyst, dentigerous
PAX	CRD	Cyst, radicular
S	DT/D	Deciduous tooth/deciduous
RX	DB	Dentinal bonding agent
PAX	DC	Dilacerated crown
PAX	DR	Dilacerated root
E	PCD	Direct pulp capping
G	D	Distal
O	EC	Elastic chain (power chain)
PA	ED	Enamel defect
PA	EH	Enamel hypocalicification/hypoplasia

Category[a]	Abbreviation	Meaning
PAX	EG	Eosinophilic granuloma
PAX	EGL	Eosinophilic granuloma lingual (tongue)
PAX	EGC	Eosinophilic granuloma lip (chelitis)
S	EP	Epulis
PA	EP	Epulis (fibrous, ossifying)
R	RL4	Extensive structure damage
S	XS	Extraction with sectioning
R	SE	Extrinsic staining (metal, etc.)
O	EXT	Extrusion
G	F	Facial
PAX	FEN	Fenestration
PAX	OM-FS	Fibrosarcoma
PAX	EP/F	Fibrous epulis
P	FAR	Flap, apically repositioning
P	FCR	Flap, coronally repositioning
P	FGG	Flap, free gingival graft
P	FLS	Flap, lateral sliding
P	FRB	Flap, reverse bevel
P	FG	Fluoride gel
P	FV	Fluoride varnish
PAX	FB	Foreign body
PA	FX	Fracture (tooth, jaw, etc.)
S	FR-P	Fracture repair—pin
S	FR-PL	Fracture repair—plate
S	FR-SC	Fracture repair—screw
S	FR-S	Fracture repair—splint
S	FR-W	Fracture repair—wire
S	FX	Fractured tooth
E	FX	Fractured tooth
PX	FRE	Frenectomy
PX	FRN	Frenotomy
P	F1	Furcation exposed
P	F2M	Furcation exposed, undermined, mesial
P	FE	Furcation exposure
P	F1F	Furcation exposure, exposed, facial
P	F3	Furcation open through to other side
P	FA	Furcation subclass A—less than 25%
P	FB	Furcation subclass B—25–50% vertical
P	FC	Furcation subclass C—greater than 50%
P	F2	Furcation undermined
PAX	EP/G	Giant cell epulis

Category[a]	Abbreviation	Meaning
PAX	GCF	Gingival crevicular fluid
PX	GCF	Gingival crevicular fluid
PX	GH	Gingival hyperplasia/hypertrophy
PX	GM	Gingival margin
PX	GR	Gingival recession
P	GV/GVP	Gingivectomy/gingivoplasty
P	GI	Gingivitis index
PAX	GLS	Glossitis
PAX	GB	Granuloma, buccal
PAX	GL	Granuloma, lingual
P	PD4	Greater than 50% attachment loss
P	GTR	Guided tissue regeneration
E	GP	Gutta percha
PAX	HT	Hairy tongue
P	IMP	Implant
O	IM	Impressions/models
G	I	Incisal or incisor
E	PCI	Indirect pulp capping
RX	IL	Inlay
S	IO	Interceptive orthodontics
O	IO	Interceptive orthodontics
O	IOD	Interceptive orthodontics, deciduous
O	IOP	Interceptive orthodontics, permanent
S	IDW	Interdental wiring
O	INT	Intrusion
P	PD2	Less than 25% attachment loss
G	L	Lingual
PAX	LG	Lingual granuloma
RX	C5	Lingual or facial, cemento-enamel junction, no pit and fissure
PAX	LM	Lingual or glossal mass
PAX	LFD	Lip fold dermatitis
PAX	LUP	Lupus erythematous
P	LPS	Lymphocytic/plasmacytic stomatitis
PAX	OM-LS	Lymphosarcoma
PAX	OM-MM	Malignant melanoma—oral mass
O	MAL	Malocclusion (modified angle class)
PAX	MN/FX	Mandibular fracture
PAX	MX/FX	Maxillary fracture
G	M	Mesial
RX	C3	Mesial or distal; incisor, no ridge

Category[a]	Abbreviation	Meaning
P	GI1	Mild inflammation; slight color change
P	PI2	Moderate accumulation of plaque
P	CI2	Moderate amount of supra- and subgingival calculus
P	GI2	Moderate inflammation; redness, edema
PA	M2	Moderate tooth mobility
G	M	Molar
PX	MGM	Mucogingival margin
PX	MM	Mucous membrane
E	NE	Near exposure
P	CI0	No calculus
P	PI0	No plaque
E	NV	Nonvital
RX	NVBL	Nonvital bleaching
P	GI0	Normal gingiva
PA	M0	Normal or no tooth mobility
G	O	Occlusal
RX	C1	Occlusal or pit and fissure; molar and premolar
G	OS	Occlusal survey
P	OP	Odontoplasty
RX	OL	Onlay
P	RPO	Open root planing
S	OM	Oral mass
PA	OM	Oral mass (malignant melanoma, squamous cell carcinoma, fibrosarcoma lymphosarcoma)
P	OAF	Oroantral fistula
S	ONF	Oronasal fistula
S	ONF/R	Oronasal fistula repair
O	OAA	Ortho appliance adjustment
O	OAI	Ortho appliance installation
O	OAR	Ortho appliance removal
O	OA	Orthodontic appliance
O	OC	Orthodontic consultation (with genetic)
O	OR	Orthodontic recheck
S	OI	Osseous implant
S	OSW	Osseous wiring
PAX	EP/O	Ossifying epulis
PAX	OST	Osteomyelitis
PAX	OM-OSC	Osteosarcoma
PAX	PT	Palatal trauma defect
S	PLT	Palate
PAX	PAP	Papillomatosis

Category[a]	Abbreviation	Meaning
PAX	PEM	Pemphigus /V—vulgaris /B—bullous
PX	W1	Perio bony pocket, 1-wall
PX	W2	Perio bony pocket, 2-wall
PX	W3	Perio bony pocket, 3-wall
PX	W4	Perio bony pocket, 4-wall "cup lesion"
PX	PG	Perio pocket, gingival (pseudopocket)
PX	PIB	Perio pocket, infrabony
PX	P7	Perio pocket, 7 mm
PX	PSB	Perio pocket, suprabony
P	PDI	Periodontal disease index
P	PDL	Periodontal ligament
PX	PP	Periodontal pocket
P	PS	Periodontal surgery
S	PT/P	Permanent tooth/permanent
RX	P&F	Pit and fissure
RX	P&FS	Pit and fissure sealant
PAX	PLQ	Plaque
PX	PLQ	Plaque
PAX	PI	Plaque index
P	PI	Plaque index (Silness and Loe)
O	PXB	Posterior cross-bite
G	PM	Premolar
O	MAL 3	Prognathia
E	PC	Pulp capping
E	PE	Pulp exposure
G	RAD	Radiograph
R	RL1	Resorptive lesion, into enamel and dentin
R	RL2	Resorptive lesion, into enamel only
R	RL3	Resorptive lesion, into root canal system
R	RL4	Resorptive lesion, portion of crown/root missing
R	RL5	Resorptive lesion, crown missing (also is RtR, retained roots)
R	R	Restoration
R	R/A	Restoration, amalgam
R	R/C	Restoration/composite
R	R/I	Restoration/glass ionomer
RX	C4	Restoration mesial-incisal distal, mesial incisal or incisal-distal, incisor with ridge
RX	C2	Restoration mesial-occlusal distal, mesial occlusal or occlusal-distal, molars and premolars
PA	RD	Retained deciduous tooth

Category[a]	Abbreviation	Meaning
S	RD	Retained deciduous tooth
S	RTR	Retained root
E	RGF	Retrograde filling
E	RGF/A	Retrograde filling—amalgam
RX	C7	Root
RX	C8	Root apex
E	RC	Root canal therapy
PX	RE	Root exposure
P	RP	Root planing
E	RRX	Root resection (hemisection)
R	RR	Root resorption
O	ROT	Rotation
PAX	SAL	Salivary gland (sublingual, mandibular, paratid, zygometic, molar [cat])
PA	2D	Secondary dentin
P	GI3	Severe inflammation; marked
PA	M3	Severe tooth mobility
S	X	Simple extraction
PA	M1	Slight tooth mobility
P	SPL	Splint
PAX	OM-SCC	Squamous cell carcinoma
R	SI	Staining, intrinsic (blood, TTC)
PAX	STM	Stomatitis
P	SC	Subgingival curettage
PAX	SL	Sublingual
PAX	SLG	Sublingual granuloma
PX	SUL	Sulcus
P	SBI	Sulcus bleeding index (1, 2, 3)
PA	SN	Supernumerary
P	CI1	Supragingival calculus extend only
S	SM	Surgery—mandibulectomy
S	SX	Surgery—maxillectomy
S	SP	Surgery—palate
S	XSS	Surgical extraction
S	SO	Surgical orthopedics
E	RCS	Surgical root canal (apicoectomy)
PAX	SYM	Symphysis
PAX	SYM/S	Symphysis separation
G	TMJ	Temporomandibular joint
PAX	TMJ/DP	Temporomandibular joint dysplasia
PAX	TMJ/FX	Temporomandibular joint fracture

Category[a]	Abbreviation	Meaning
PAX	TMJ/L	Temporomandibular joint luxation
P	PI1	Thin film along gingival margin
P	F3FA	Through exposure, facial, less than 25%
O	TIP	Tipping
PA	TA	Tooth avulsed
PA	TL	Tooth luxated
E	TRX	Tooth resection (hemisection)
G	TN	Treatment needed
G	TP	Treatment plan
E	TP	Treatment planning
P	TP	Treatment planning
RX	VER	Veneer
RX	VBL	Vital bleaching
E	VP	Vital pulpotomy
E	VT	Vital tooth or pulp
PAX	VWD	von Willebrand's disease
S	WIR	Wiring
O	WRY	Wry mouth
E	ZOE	Zinc oxide/eugenol

[a]Categories for abbreviations:

E = endodontics, G = general terminology,
M = miscellaneous, O = orthodontics, P = periodontics, PA = pathology,
R = restoratives, S = oral surgery.

"Extended" categories for abbreviations less frequently used:

PAX = pathology, extended, PX = periodontics, extended, and
RX = restoratives, extended.

Position Statement of the American Veterinary Dental College

American Veterinary Dental College's position statement regarding veterinary dental health care providers

The American Veterinary Dental College (AVDC) has developed the following position as a means to safeguard veterinary dental patients and ensure the qualifications of persons performing veterinary dental procedures.

Primary Responsibility for Veterinary Dental Care

The AVDC defines veterinary dentistry as the art and practice of oral health care in animals other than people. It is a discipline of veterinary medicine and surgery. Diagnosis, treatment, and management of veterinary oral health care are to be provided and supervised by licensed veterinarians or by veterinarians working within a university or industry.

Who May Provide Veterinarian-Supervised Dental Health Care

The AVDC accepts that the following health care workers may assist responsible veterinarians in dental procedures or actually perform dental prophylactic services while under direct, in-room supervision by a veterinarian if permitted by local law: licensed, certified, or registered veterinary technicians; veterinary assistants with advanced dental training; dentists; and registered dental hygienists.

Operative Dentistry and Oral Surgery

The AVDC considers operative dentistry to be any dental procedure that invades the hard or soft oral tissues including, but not limited to, a procedure that alters the structure of one or more teeth or repairs damaged and diseased teeth. Veterinarians should perform operative dentistry and oral surgery.

Extraction of Teeth

The AVDC considers extraction of teeth to be included in the practice of veterinary dentistry. Decision making is the responsibility of veterinarians, with the consent of pet owners, when electing to extract teeth. Only veterinarians shall determine which teeth are to be extracted and perform extraction procedures.

Tasks That May Be Performed by Veterinary Technicians

The AVDC considers it appropriate for veterinarians to delegate maintenance dental care and certain dental tasks to veterinary technicians. Tasks appropriately performed by veterinary technicians include dental prophylaxis and certain procedures that do not result in alterations in the shape, structure, or positional location of teeth in the dental arch. A veterinar-

ian may direct a technician to perform these tasks providing that the veterinarian is physically present and supervising the treatment and providing that the technician has received appropriate training.

The AVDC supports advanced training of veterinary technicians to perform additional ancillary dental services (eg, taking impressions, making models, charting veterinary dental lesions, taking and developing dental radiographs, performing nonsurgical subgingival root scaling and debridement) providing that they do not alter the structure of the tooth.

Tasks That May Be Performed by Veterinary Assistants (Not Registered, Certified, or Licensed)

The AVDC supports appropriate training of veterinary assistants to perform the following dental services: supragingival scaling and polishing, taking and developing dental radiographs, making impressions, and making models.

Tasks That May Be Performed by Dentists, Registered Dental Hygienists, and Other Dental Health Care Providers

The AVDC recognizes that dentists, registered dental hygienists, and other dental health care providers in good standing may perform those procedures for which they have been qualified under the direct supervision of a veterinarian. The supervising veterinarian will be responsible for the welfare of the patient and any treatment performed on the patient.

Endorsement of 1996 American Association of Equine Practitioners' Position Statement on Equine Dentistry

The AVDC endorses the following position statement adopted by the American Association of Equine Practitioners in October 1996:

> Equine dentistry is the practice of veterinary medicine and should not be performed by anyone other than a licensed veterinarian or a certified veterinary technician under the employ of a licensed veterinarian. Any dental activity requiring sedation, tranquilization, analgesia or anesthesia, and procedures which are invasive of the tissue of the oral cavity, including but not limited to extraction of teeth, amputation of large molar, incisor or canine teeth, the extraction of first premolar teeth (wolf teeth) and repair of damaged or diseased teeth, must be performed by a veterinarian. The rasping (floating) of molar, premolar and canine teeth and the removal of deciduous incisor and premolar teeth (caps) may, provided a valid veterinarian-client-patient relationship exists, be performed by a certified veterinary technician under the employ of a veterinarian.

The AVDC understands that individual states have regulations that govern the practice of veterinary medicine. This position statement is intended to be a model for veterinary dental practice and does not replace existing laws.

Adopted by the American Veterinary Dental College, Apr 5, 1998. For more information, contact Dr. Frank J. M. Verstraete, Secretary, American Veterinary Dental College, Department of Surgical and Radiological Sciences, School of Veterinary Medicine, University of California, Davis, CA 95616.
Opinions expressed are not necessarily those of the AVMA.

Dental Suppliers

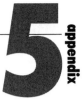

The following companies and individuals are frequent advertisers in the *Journal of Veterinary Dentistry*:

General Equipment and Supplies

Cislak Instruments, Inc.
1-847-729-2904
1-847-729-2447 Fax

Dr. Shipp's Laboratories
1-310-550-0107
1-310-550-1664 Fax
DrShipp@worldnet.att.net

Henry Schein (most complete range of products)
1-800-872-4346 (1-800-V-SCHEIN)
1-800-483-8329 (1-800-4-VET-FAX) Fax
www.henryschein.com

Oral Health Products

Addison Laboratories, Inc.
1-800-331-2530

Allerderm-Virbac, Inc.
1-800-338-3659

Heska
1-800-404-3752 (1-800-GO-HESKA)
www.heska.com

Nylabone Corporation
1-732-988-5466 Fax

VRx, Inc.
1-800-969-7387
VRxProduct@aol.com

Orthodontic Appliances and Crowns

Veterinary Dental Laboratory of America
1-814-474-5806
1-814-474-3241 Fax
74253656@compuserve.com

Dental Equipment Repair

CBI (C. Brungart, Inc.).
1-800-654-5705

Dental Diets

Hills Prescription Diets
(sponsor of Pet Dental Health Month)
1-800-354-4557

Dental Pharmaceuticals

Pfizer
www.pfizer.com/ah

Pharmacia & Upjohn Co.
1-800-394-6292

Index